THE SHATTERED MIRROR

Portraits of Childhood and the Architecture of War

This is dedicated to the children lost their lives in these devastating wars. Your have suffered in an earthly inhumane way, but you are now in the arms of your Lord.

CONTENTS

Title Page
Dedication
CHAPTER 1: The Vertical Siege — 1
CHAPTER 2: The Subterranean Nursery — 7
CHAPTER 3: The Boy Who Walked Into the Void — 16
CHAPTER 4: The Hands That Break the Stones — 24
CHAPTER 5: The Art of Kintsugi — 30
 The Architects of Tomorrow — 39
 PART II: THE EROSION — 45
CHAPTER 6: The Classroom of Dust — 46
CHAPTER 7: The Cold Concrete (Ukraine) — 53
CHAPTER 8: The Wolf of the Camp — 57
CHAPTER 9: The Algorithm of Fear (Gaza) — 66
CHAPTER 10: The Iron Puberty — 70
CHAPTER 11: The Glass Wall (Ukraine) — 77
CHAPTER 12: The Shrinking World — 81
CHAPTER 13: The Chemistry of the Soldier — 86
CHAPTER 14: The Classroom of Revenge — 90
PART III: THE RECLAMATION — 94
CHAPTER 15: The Un-Doing — 95
CHAPTER 16: The Defrosting — 101

CHAPTER 17: The Mosaic 106

SELECTED BIBLIOGRAPHY 109

Introduction

The human brain is not designed for the infinite present. It is built to categorize time into a comforting rhythm of *before*, *during*, and *after*. We endure a crisis because we believe in the "after."

But for a child born into the generational conflicts of the twenty-first century, there is no "after." There is only the "during."

When a seven-year-old in Gaza hears the low-frequency hum of a surveillance drone, her cortisol levels do not spike and return to baseline, as biology dictates they should. They remain elevated, a high-water mark that never recedes. When a boy in the eastern Democratic Republic of Congo learns to distinguish the snap of a twig from the click of a rifle safety, his neural pathways are actively pruning away the ability to learn algebra or trust a neighbor, prioritizing instead the singular, ancient imperative of survival.

This is not merely a story of sadness. It is a story of **biological renovation**.

War is often measured in the geometry of destruction: the tonnage of rubble, the radius of a blast, the shifting lines on a map. But the most permanent landscape of war is the internal one. Violence enters the child through the eyes and ears, but it settles in the marrow. It rewires the architecture of the mind. It alters the expression of genes. It turns the body's own defense systems into a chronic siege engine.

The Geography of Trauma

This book is an expedition into that internal landscape. To understand it, we must travel to the places where childhood has been suspended.

We will go to **Sudan**, where the displacement of millions has created a psychological void—a generation growing up without the "mirror" of community to tell them who they are. We will walk the streets of **Kharkiv, Ukraine**, to understand the auditory trauma of air raid sirens and how the loss of "safe sound" shatters a child's capacity for deep sleep and memory consolidation. We will enter the dense, complex history of the **Congo**, to witness the moral injury of children forced to become perpetrators of the very violence they fled. And we will look unflinchingly at **Palestine**, specifically Gaza, to study the effects of confinement and continuous traumatic stress, where the horizon itself is a barrier.

These regions differ in politics, terrain, and language. But the children inhabiting them share a common dialect: the neurobiology of threat.

Beyond the Statistics

You likely picked up this book because the numbers have become numbing. The United Nations releases reports, the Red Cross issues warnings, and the statistics blur into a monolithic tragedy. "One million children." "Five hundred thousand displaced." The human mind cannot empathize with a million; it shuts down. It can only empathize with one.

Therefore, this book is not a catalogue of misery. It is a collection of portraits.

We will follow individual lives—anonymized to protect them, but rigorously detailed. You will see how they play, how they dream, and how they hide. We will place these narratives alongside the latest clinical research in **epigenetics, neuroplasticity, and developmental psychology**. We will ask: What happens to a developing frontal cortex when it is bathed in adrenaline for five years? How does a child construct a concept of "good" and "evil" when the adults around them have lost control of the world?

The Mirror

The title of this book, *The Shattered Mirror*, refers to the psychological concept of "mirroring." A child learns they exist, and that they are good, by seeing themselves reflected in the eyes of a loving, safe caregiver. War shatters that mirror. Parents, consumed by their own terror and grief, often cannot provide that reflection. The environment reflects only danger. The child looks out at the world and sees no reflection of their own humanity.

And yet, the most shocking discovery you will make in these pages is not the fragility of these children, but their terrifying adaptability. The brain is plastic; it molds to fit its container. These children are adapting to their hells with genius precision. The tragedy is that the very adaptations that keep them alive in war —hyper-vigilance, dissociation, aggression—are the very things that will make peace, if it ever comes, a foreign and difficult country.

This is not a book about the past. It is a book about the future. The children of Sudan, Gaza, Ukraine, and Congo are the future architects of their nations. If we wish to know what those nations will look like in twenty years, we must look at the blueprints currently being drawn inside the minds of their children.

Let us begin.

CHAPTER 1: THE VERTICAL SIEGE

Location: Gaza Strip
Subject: Tariq, Age 9
Clinical Focus: Allostatic Load and the Erasure of Safe Space

The air in Gaza has a texture. It is not merely oxygen and nitrogen; it is a suspension of pulverized concrete, diesel fumes, and the metallic alkalinity of old rebar. For nine-year-old Tariq, living in a dense neighborhood north of Rafah, the act of breathing is a sensory reminder of where he is. But it is the sound that defines his existence.

In the lexicon of modern warfare, we talk about "the front line." We imagine a horizontal boundary: soldiers on one side, enemies on the other. But for Tariq, there is no horizontal front line. The threat is vertical. It hangs above him, a permanent, invisible ceiling of surveillance and potential obliteration.

It is 6:00 AM. The sun has not yet crested the shattered skyline, but the "Zanana" is already awake. *Zanana* is the street name the children of Gaza have given to the Israeli surveillance drones. It translates roughly to "the buzzing" or "the nagging wife." It is a low, glottal hum, like a lawnmower running three streets away, but it never stops. It is omnipresent.

Tariq wakes up on a mattress shared with his two younger

brothers. He does not stretch. He does not yawn. His eyes open, and his body goes rigid. This is the first psychological casualty of the war: the loss of the "hypnagogic transition." Most children drift slowly from sleep to wakefulness. Tariq snaps into consciousness. His brain has learned that vulnerability is fatal.

He listens. He is performing a complex auditory calculus, filtering the background hum of the drone to detect anomalies—the whistle of a falling projectile, the roar of a jet, the crumble of a nearby structure.

The house is silent. His mother is boiling water. The sound of the kettle is domestic, normal. It is this juxtaposition—the domestic interior against the hostile exterior—that creates a cognitive dissonance so severe it fractures the developing mind.

The Biology of the "Always-On"

To understand what is happening inside Tariq's body at 6:05 AM, we must look at the **HPA Axis (Hypothalamic-Pituitary-Adrenal Axis)**.

In a healthy human, a threat triggers the amygdala (the brain's smoke detector). The amygdala sends a distress signal to the hypothalamus, which activates the sympathetic nervous system. The adrenal glands dump adrenaline and cortisol into the bloodstream. The heart races, blood moves from digestion to the muscles, and the body prepares to fight or flee. Once the threat passes, the parasympathetic nervous system engages the "brake," and cortisol levels drop.

For Tariq, the brake is broken.

Because the drone is always overhead, the threat never passes. Tariq is living in a state of **Chronic Hyper-arousal**. His baseline cortisol levels are permanently elevated. He is marinating in stress hormones.

Dr. Samah Jabr, a leading psychiatrist in the West Bank, has noted that in this context, the term PTSD (Post-Traumatic Stress Disorder) is clinically inaccurate. There is no "Post." The trauma is repetitive and continuous. The medical community is shifting toward a new diagnosis for children in these zones: **Continuous Traumatic Stress (CTS)**.

Under CTS, the body begins to attack itself. The constant flood of cortisol suppresses Tariq's immune system. He is smaller than an average nine-year-old. He suffers from skin rashes that refuse to heal. His body is diverting every ounce of metabolic energy toward survival, leaving nothing for growth or repair. He is biologically weathering, aging on a cellular level at twice the rate of a child in London or New York.

The Geography of Containment

Tariq steps outside to fetch water. The street is a canyon of grey.

The psychological impact of Gaza is unique because of the **claustrophobia of war**. In Ukraine, millions of mothers and children fled across the border to Poland or Romania. It was a trauma of displacement, yes, but it offered an escape valve. In Sudan, families flee into the bush.
In Gaza, the borders are sealed. To the west, the sea is patrolled. To the north, east, and south, fences and walls. The sky is occupied.

This creates a phenomenon known as **Learned Helplessness**, a theory originally developed by Martin Seligman. When a subject learns that no action they take can alter the outcome of an aversive event, they stop trying. They become passive.
But Tariq is not passive; he is manic. He runs to the water truck. He fights for a place in line. This is the paradox of the besieged child: they oscillate between total despair and aggressive hyperactivity.

"Move," he snaps at a smaller boy, shoving him. The boy shoves back. A fistfight breaks out.

This aggression is not malice. It is a discharge. Tariq has nowhere to run and nowhere to hide, so the adrenaline trapped in his muscles must find an exit. Violence becomes a language of release. The social fabric among children begins to fray. In a normal childhood, play is a rehearsal for adult life. In the siege, play becomes a rehearsal for combat.

The Event

At 2:00 PM, the hum of the Zanana changes pitch. It is joined by the deeper, tearing sound of an F-16 jet.

Tariq is playing marbles in the alley. The sound is the cue. It happens in milliseconds. The air pressure drops—a physical sensation of a vacuum being created. Then, the earth jumps.

It is not a sound at first. It is a concussion. The blast wave hits Tariq's chest before the noise reaches his ears. He is thrown backward against a cinderblock wall.

Then comes the sound: a cracking, apocalyptic thunder that seems to originate from inside his own skull.

He does not scream. He goes silent. This is **Dissociation**.
When the reality is too terrible to be processed, the brain pulls the plug on the conscious mind. Tariq's eyes are open, but he is not "there." He is watching the scene from a distance, through the wrong end of a telescope. He sees the dust rising like a phantom. He sees a neighbor screaming, but the audio track has been severed.

This dissociation is a brilliant survival mechanism. It acts as a chemical anesthetic. If he were fully present, the terror might stop his heart. So, his brain severs the connection between emotion and memory.

However, the cost is high. When children dissociate frequently, their memory becomes fragmented. They lose the narrative of their own lives. They cannot recall what happened yesterday, or they remember it in disjointed flashes—a color, a smell, a sound— without a coherent story. Tariq is losing his autobiography.

The Ruins of Sleep

Night falls. The electricity is out, as it usually is. The darkness is total, save for the flashes of artillery on the horizon.

Tariq lies on the mattress. This is the hardest time. During the day, the cortex (the thinking brain) can exert some control. At night, the cortex goes offline, and the primitive brain takes over.

He closes his eyes, and the "movies" start. This is what the children call flashbacks. They are not memories; they are re-experiences. He smells the sulfur. He feels the wall against his back.

He wets the bed.

At nine years old, this is a source of profound shame. He hides the wet patch, pulling the blanket over it. Enuresis (bed-wetting) is epidemic among children in conflict zones. It is a sign of **Regressive Behavior**. Under extreme stress, the psyche retreats to an earlier developmental stage where it felt safer. Tariq, the tough boy who shoves kids in the water line, returns to toddlerhood in the dark.

He lies awake, listening to the Zanana. It is watching him. He knows it can see body heat. He wonders if his heat looks different because he is afraid.

He pulls his knees to his chest. He is waiting for the morning, but he does not believe in the morning. He only believes in the night.

This is the architecture of the siege. It is not just the walls around the city; it is the wall built around the heart. Tariq is still alive. He has all his limbs. He has no shrapnel in his skin. But the war has already taken him. It has taken his sleep, his trust, his biology, and his future.

He is a veteran at nine. And the war has not yet ended.

CHAPTER 2: THE SUBTERRANEAN NURSERY

Location: Kharkiv, Ukraine

Subject: Olena, Age 6

Clinical Focus: Acoustic Trauma, Sleep Architecture, and the Loss of Sanctuary

I. The Frequency of Dread

In Kharkiv, the war does not begin with an explosion. It begins with a frequency.

It starts as a low moan from the city's industrial speakers, mounted on rooftops that used to look over coffee shops and parks. The sound rises—a mechanical, undulating wail that hits a specific pitch designed during the Cold War to bypass the logic centers of the human cortex and vibrate the brainstem directly. It is a sound that does not ask for attention; it commandeers the nervous system. It says, in a language older than words: *The sky is no longer yours.*

For six-year-old Olena, the sound is the conductor of her life. She is sitting on the floor of her apartment's hallway, the "two-wall rule" sanctuary where the glass from the windows cannot reach her. She is playing with a plastic horse. When the siren begins, she does not cry. She does not look to her mother for confirmation. She simply stops playing.

Her pupils dilate. Her breathing arrests. This is the **Orienting Response**, the biological pivot from safety to survival. In a healthy child, this response is rare. In Olena, it is a daily rhythm.

She stands up and walks to the front door. There is a backpack there, pre-packed with a grim, adult efficiency: a stuffed rabbit named 'Zayats,' a flashlight, a juice box, wet wipes, and a laminated card pinned to the inside pocket listing her blood type and her grandmother's phone number.

"Boots," her mother, Iryna, says. Her voice is tight, a wire pulled to the breaking point.

Olena puts on her boots. They do not run. Running implies panic, and panic is dangerous. They move with the heavy, frantic precision of people who have done this a hundred times. They step out into the stairwell. The elevator is a death trap, so they walk down nine flights of concrete stairs.

Outside, the air is biting. It is February in Eastern Europe. The sky is a flat, indifferent grey. The city is strangely silent, save for the wail. It is a "ghost city" silence—the suspension of life before the strike.

They hurry toward the metro station entrance, a concrete mouth in the pavement. As they cross the street, a sonic boom cracks the air—a jet breaking the sound barrier invisible above the cloud layer. Olena flinches. It is a full-body convulsion, a **myoclonic jerk**. Her hands fly up to cover her ears, and she crouches.
This is not a choice. It is a reflex arc that has been burned into her neural pathways. The auditory cortex has become a threat-detection center. The wind, a slamming door, a car backfiring —they are no longer neutral sounds. They are preludes to annihilation.

II. The Descent

The Kharkiv Metro is a monument to Soviet paranoia, dug deep enough to withstand a nuclear first strike. To enter it is to travel down a steep, mechanical throat into the belly of the earth.

As Olena steps onto the escalator, the sensory world shifts violently. The cold bite of the winter air vanishes, replaced by a stagnant, recycled warmth. The smell changes. The scent of snow and exhaust gives way to the subterranean perfume: ozone, damp wool, granite dust, unwashed bodies, and the metallic tang of old electricity.

The descent takes two full minutes. It is a journey between worlds.

Above, there is the unpredictable geometry of shrapnel. Below, there is the crushing stability of granite. As they descend, the noise of the siren fades, replaced by a low, human hum. It is the sound of two thousand people breathing in a confined space.

They step off the escalator onto the platform of the Heroiv Pratsi station.

It was once a cathedral of transit—high vaulted ceilings, marble columns, chandeliers. Now, it is a refugee camp frozen in marble. Tents are pitched in chaotic rows. Camping mattresses form a patchwork quilt over the cold stone. Clotheslines are strung between the pillars, drying socks and underwear in the stagnant air.

This is the **Static Village**.

"Home," Olena whispers, though she doesn't mean it.

They find their spot—Section 4, near the vending machines. Their "apartment" is a yoga mat and two sleeping bags. Their neighbors are the Volkovs, an elderly couple who sleep sitting up, and a teenager named Dima who stares at his phone, his face illuminated by the blue light of the screen, scrolling through Telegram channels for news of rocket strikes.

Olena takes off her boots. She places Zayats, the rabbit, on the pillow. She creates a boundary. This mat is hers. Everything outside the mat is chaos.

III. The Dyadic Failure

Iryna sits down heavily. She pulls out her phone. Her thumb moves in a blur.

This is the most critical variable in the equation of Olena's trauma: **The Primary Caregiver**.

Donald Winnicott, the 20th-century pediatrician and psychoanalyst, introduced the concept of the "holding environment." A child creates their reality through the parent. If the mother is calm, the world is safe. If the mother is terrified, the world is ending. The parent acts as an external nervous system, regulating the child's heartbeat with their own.

But Iryna cannot hold Olena. Iryna is shattering.

Her husband, Olena's father, is in the Donbas region. He hasn't messaged in twelve hours. Iryna is checking the "Last Seen" timestamp on WhatsApp. She is vibrating with cortisol.

Olena crawls into Iryna's lap. She needs "co-regulation." She needs her mother's heartbeat to be slow and steady. But what she finds is a racing pulse and shallow breathing. She smells the "fear pheromones" in her mother's sweat—a distinct, acidic chemical signal that humans emit when under mortal threat.

Olena pulls back. She cannot find safety here.

"Mama?"

"Hush, Olena. Not now. I'm reading."

The rejection is not malicious; Iryna is simply at capacity. But for Olena, it confirms a terrifying truth: *The adults have lost control.* The captains of the ship are panic-stricken.
This creates **Dyadic Dysregulation**. The anxiety bounces back and forth between mother and daughter, amplifying like a microphone placed too close to a speaker. A feedback loop of terror.

IV. The Architecture of Ruined Sleep

Time in the metro is a blur. There is no sun to mark the passage of day to night. There are only the fluorescent lights, which are dimmed but never extinguished.

Night falls on the surface, but down here, it is just "Quiet Time." The station settles into a restless, collective tossing.

Olena lies in her sleeping bag. This is the battlefield of the mind.

Sleep is not merely rest; it is a neurological construction site.

Specifically, **REM (Rapid Eye Movement)** sleep is the phase where the brain processes emotions. It takes the terror of the day—the siren, the boom—and strips the visceral emotion from the memory, filing it away as "the past." It is a cleansing mechanism. But you cannot enter deep REM sleep if you do not feel safe. The brain remains in "sentinel mode," keeping the sensory channels open for danger.

Olena drifts off. Twenty minutes later, the ground vibrates. A train, used for maintenance or moving supplies deeper into the tunnel, rumbles past on the far track.

Olena's eyes snap open. She gasps, sitting bolt upright.

She has not completed a sleep cycle. She is stuck in **Stage 1 and 2** —light sleep. She is missing the restorative, emotional healing of deep sleep.

This is **Sleep Fragmentation**.

Without REM, the amygdala (the brain's emotional center) becomes hyper-active, and the prefrontal cortex (the logic center) becomes sluggish. A child deprived of REM sleep is an emotional raw nerve. They cannot regulate their temper. They cannot focus. They are chemically unbalanced.

Olena looks at the ceiling. She sees patterns in the marble. She imagines they are faces. Monsters. She wets herself.

The warmth spreads in the sleeping bag. The shame follows instantly. She is six; she stopped wetting the bed three years ago. But under extreme stress, the psyche retreats. It goes back to a time of dependency. This is **Regression**.

She does not wake her mother. She lies in the damp cold, shivering, punishing herself for a biological failure she cannot control. She stares at the fluorescent light, waiting for a morning she will not see.

V. The School in the Iron Belly

"Wake up, little ones. School time."

A volunteer named Sveta walks through the rows of sleeping bags, clapping her hands. Sveta was a university professor before the war. Now she is the headmistress of Platform 4.

The "school" is a stationary metro car parked permanently on the third track. The children climb inside. The seats are the desks. The windows, looking out into the black tunnel, are the walls.

Olena sits next to a boy named Maxim. Maxim is eight. He has stopped speaking. He hasn't said a word since a shell hit his apartment block in Saltivka. He communicates only by pushing things away or pulling them closer.

Sveta hands out paper and crayons. "Today," she says brightly, "draw your favorite place."

The children bend over their papers. The air in the car is stuffy, smelling of old upholstery.

Olena draws. She presses the wax crayon hard against the paper.

She draws a house. But she draws it underground. She draws a thick black line above the roof.

"What is that?" Sveta asks, crouching beside her.

"The ground," Olena says.

"And where is the sun?"

"It's broken," Olena says. She picks up a black crayon and scribbles over the top half of the page. "The sky is bad."

This is the **Cognitive Remapping** of the world. In Olena's developing brain, the concepts of "Light," "Sky," and "Outside" are being re-categorized from *Good* to *Threat*. Conversely, "Dark," "Underground," and "Confined" are being re-categorized as *Safety*.

She is becoming a creature of the dark.

Suddenly, a loud *clank* echoes through the tunnel—a metal pipe falling in a maintenance shaft.
The reaction in the train car is instantaneous. It is not chaos; it is silence. Every child freezes. Twenty heads snap toward the sound. Maxim dives under the seat. Olena drops her crayon and covers her neck with her hands.

It is a synchronized ballet of trauma. These children are no longer individuals; they are a flock, moving in unison to the predator's rhythm.

Sveta waits. She does not tell them "it's okay," because she knows they won't believe her. She waits for their nervous systems to verify the threat level.

"Just a pipe," Sveta says softly. "Just a pipe. Breathe."

Olena slowly lowers her hands. But the adrenaline is already in her blood. Her hands are shaking. She cannot hold the crayon anymore. She stares at her drawing of the black sun.

VI. The Ghost of the Future

Later that afternoon, a rumor ripples through the station. *The bombing has stopped. The shops are open for an hour.*
Iryna grabs Olena's hand. "We need fresh air. We need to go up."

Olena resists. She plants her feet. "No."

"Olena, we need food. Come."

They ride the escalator up. The ascent is terrifying. As they near the surface, the light grows brighter—a harsh, white winter glare. Olena squints. Her eyes, adapted to the gloom, burn.

They step out into the street. The silence is profound. The snow is pristine, white and sparkling. But across the street, the administration building is gone. It is simply not there. In its place is a hollowed-out tooth of concrete and twisted steel.

Olena looks at the ruin. She looks at the sky. It is blue, vast, and terrifyingly open. There is no ceiling. There is nothing to stop the falling.

She feels a wave of vertigo. This is **Agoraphobia** induced by war. The open space feels like a nakedness.
"Let's go back," she whispers. "Mama, let's go back."

"Just a minute," Iryna says, breathing in the cold air, closing her eyes. She is desperate for the sky.

But Olena is pulling at her hand, dragging her toward the black mouth of the metro. She wants the stone. She wants the weight of the earth above her head. She wants the tomb, because the tomb is the only place that feels like a womb.

"Please," Olena begs, and a tear finally leaks out. "The sky will kill us."

Iryna looks down at her daughter. She sees the terror in her eyes —a terror that is not just of the bombs, but of the world itself. She realizes then that the war has done something worse than destroy their home. It has destroyed her daughter's ability to love the light.

"Okay," Iryna says, her voice breaking. "Okay. We go down."

They turn their backs on the sun and descend, back into the twilight, back to the static village, where the air is stale and safe, and where the only dreams are the ones that happen when you are awake.

CHAPTER 3: THE BOY WHO WALKED INTO THE VOID

Location: The Road to Adré (Sudan-Chad Border)
Subject: Adil, Age 11
Clinical Focus: Ambiguous Loss, Resource Trauma, and the Dissolution of Identity

I. The Geography of Nowhere

If Ukraine is a trauma of *containment*, Sudan is a trauma of *exposure*.
For Adil, eleven years old and formerly a student of mathematics in Khartoum, the world has lost its walls. There are no bedrooms, no classrooms, no fences. There is only the horizon.

He is walking. He has been walking for nineteen days. The landscape around him is a flat, searing anvil of scrubland and red dust. The sun here is not a celestial body; it is a physical weight that sits on the back of his neck, pressing him into the earth.

In Khartoum, Adil was defined by coordinates. He was the boy who lived on Nile Street. He was the goalkeeper for the neighborhood football team. He was the son of a pharmacist.

Now, he is a coordinate in motion. He is one of the four million. As he walks, the layers of his identity are being stripped away by the wind and the heat, leaving only the biological imperative: *Move*.
He carries a plastic jerrycan. It is empty. The sound of the empty plastic banging against his thigh is the metronome of his migration. *Thump. Thump. Thump.*

II. The Psychology of Scarcity

To understand Adil's mind at this moment, we must suspend our modern understanding of "stress" and look at the **Neurobiology of Scarcity**.
In a stable society, the human brain operates heavily in the **Prefrontal Cortex**. This is the seat of executive function: planning, empathy, abstract thought, and future-orientation.
But Adil hasn't eaten a full meal in six days. He has had only sips of brown, tepid water.

When the body enters a state of caloric and hydrational deficit,

the brain makes a brutal economic decision. It cuts power to the "expensive" machinery (the Prefrontal Cortex) and diverts all energy to the **Limbic System** and the **Brainstem**.
Adil is no longer thinking about his math homework or his favorite team. Those neural circuits have gone dark. He is operating on "Lizard Logic." His world has shrunk to a three-foot radius around his body. He looks at the ground, scanning for three things:

1. Something wet.
2. Something edible.
3. Something sharp (danger).

This is **Cognitive Tunneling**. The periphery vanishes. Empathy vanishes. Yesterday, he saw an old woman fall by the side of the road. In Khartoum, he would have rushed to help. Here, he walked past. He did not feel guilt. He felt nothing. His brain could not afford the caloric cost of compassion.

III. The Terror of the Checkpoint

The column of refugees slows. A ripple of tension moves through the crowd, faster than a shout.

"Men with guns," someone whispers.

It is the Rapid Support Forces (RSF). They have set up a checkpoint—a rope strung across the dust, a pickup truck with a mounted machine gun, and three young men in turbans holding Kalashnikovs.

This is the flashpoint of the Sudanese trauma. In Gaza, the enemy is often distant—a drone, a jet. Here, the violence is intimate. It has a face.

Adil freezes. His mother, Fatima, grabs his shoulder. Her grip is bruising.

"Look down," she hisses. "Do not look at their eyes. Make yourself small."

Adil shrinks. This is a survival posture known as **Appeasement**.

One of the soldiers approaches. He is young, perhaps only five years older than Adil. He is chewing khat. He looks bored. He points the barrel of his rifle at Adil's chest, using it like a finger to push him back.

"What is in the can?" the soldier asks.

"Air," Adil says. His voice is a croak.

The soldier laughs. He kicks the can from Adil's hand. It skitters across the road.

"Go," the soldier says. "Run before I change my mind."

They walk. They do not run, because running provokes the predator instinct. They walk with agonizing slowness until they are out of sight. Only then does Adil vomit dry bile into the dust.

IV. Ambiguous Loss

The most profound psychological wound Adil carries is not the hunger. It is the **Question Mark**.

Nineteen days ago, when the shelling started in their neighborhood, his father, Ibrahim, went to the pharmacy to get insulin for Adil's grandmother. He said, "I will be back in ten minutes."

He never came back.

They waited for two days. Then the house next door was vaporized, and they had to leave.

Adil does not know if his father is dead. He does not know if he is alive. He does not know if he is captured.

This clinical phenomenon is called **Ambiguous Loss**, a term coined by Dr. Pauline Boss. It is widely considered the most difficult type of trauma to treat because there is no closure.
If his father were dead, Adil could grieve. There would be a body, a funeral, a "before" and an "after." But with Ambiguous Loss, the grief process is frozen. The brain cannot categorize the person. Is Ibrahim a "memory" or a "hope"?

Adil keeps a conversation running in his head.

Maybe he is at the border waiting for us.

Maybe he is in Egypt.

Maybe he is walking behind us right now.

This constant ruminating requires immense mental energy. It prevents Adil from accepting his new reality. He is living in the conditional tense. He scans every face in the miles-long column of refugees, looking for the familiar tilt of his father's shoulders. Every stranger is a potential father, and every disappointment is a fresh micro-trauma.

V. The Void of the Camp

On the twentieth day, the horizon changes. The scrubland gives way to a sea of white plastic.

They have reached Adré, on the Chad border.

It is not a city. It is a sprawl of humanitarian geometry. Tens of thousands of white tarp tents stretch as far as the eye can see. There are no trees. There is no shade. Just the blinding white of the UN logos and the red dust.

They are processed. They are given a ration card. They are given a tent—Section D, Row 41.

Adil sits inside the tent. It is 45 degrees Celsius (113°F) inside. The air smells of latrines and heated plastic.

This is the moment the adrenaline crashes. For twenty days, the journey kept him alive. The *goal* kept him alive. Now, the goal is achieved. He is "safe."
And this is when the depression hits.

In psychology, we talk about **Maslow's Hierarchy of Needs**. Adil has plummeted to the very bottom.

- **Self-Actualization:** Gone.
- **Esteem:** Gone.
- **Belonging:** Gone.
- **Safety:** Tenuous.
- **Physiological:** Barely met.

He looks at his hands. They are covered in a layer of grime that feels like a second skin. He tries to remember his bedroom in Khartoum. He tries to remember the poster of Mohamed Salah on his wall. He tries to remember the smell of his father's cologne.

But the memories are slippery. The **Hippocampus**—the brain's librarian—is struggling. The stress hormones have been so high for so long that they are actually toxic to hippocampal neurons. Adil is experiencing **Traumatic Amnesia**. The specifics of his past are fading, replaced by the overwhelming sensory input of the present: the heat, the flies, the smell.

VI. The Erasure of the Self

A week passes. Adil joins a group of boys sitting in the shade of a water truck.

They do not play football. They do not talk about school. They sit in silence, drawing lines in the dust with sticks.

"What is your name?" a boy asks.

"Adil."

"Where are you from?"

Adil hesitates. "Khartoum."

"That is gone," the boy says simply. "We are from Here now."

Adil looks at the white tents. He looks at the thousands of people who look exactly like him—dusty, thin, waiting.

This is the final tragedy of the Void. It strips you of your individuality. To the aid workers, Adil is a number on a spreadsheet. To the world, he is a "refugee." To the soldiers, he is a target.

He is losing the "I."

That night, Adil dreams. In the dream, he is back in Khartoum. The Nile is blue and cool. His father is there, laughing, holding a glass of juice.

"Drink," his father says.

Adil reaches for the glass. But just as his fingers touch the cold condensation, the siren sounds. The glass shatters. The Nile turns to dust.

Adil wakes up. He is gasping. He is in the white tent. The heat is suffocating.

He touches his face. He is crying. But he wipes the tears away quickly. In the Void, tears are a waste of water.

He lies back down and stares at the plastic ceiling, listening to the coughing of ten thousand strangers, waiting for the sun to rise and punish them all over again.

CHAPTER 4: THE HANDS THAT BREAK THE STONES

Location: North Kivu, Democratic Republic of Congo
Subject: Michel, Age 13
Clinical Focus: Moral Injury, Toxic Shame, and the Internalization of the Aggressor

I. The Green Silence

To enter the Kivu region is to enter a paradise that has been weaponized. The hills are a lush, prehistoric green, rolling under mists that smell of rain and rich, volcanic soil. It is a landscape of aggressive fertility.

But for thirteen-year-old Michel, the green is not beautiful. It is a prison wall.

He stands knee-deep in a pit of red mud. It is raining—a warm, heavy equatorial downpour that turns the earth into a slurry. He is not alone. Around him, fifty other boys, some as young as seven, are bent double, their spines curving like question marks. They are the "creuseurs"—the diggers.

They are not digging for gold. They are digging for a dull, black, heavy stone called coltan.

Michel holds a rusted rebar spike. He slams it into the clay wall of the pit. *Thwack.* He pulls. *Thwack.* He pulls.
His hands are no longer the hands of a child. The palms are calloused into leather. The fingernails are gone, worn away by the grit. But the physical deformity is secondary to the psychological one. Michel works in silence. The mine is loud—the sound of metal on stone, the shouting of the *commandants*—but the boys themselves are silent. They have learned that visibility is dangerous. To speak is to be noticed. To be noticed is to be punished.

II. The Commodity Chain

Michel does not know what coltan is. He does not know that when refined into tantalum, it becomes the heat-resistant powder that allows a smartphone to hold a charge. He does not know that the device you are likely holding to read this chapter contains a microscopic piece of the stone he is currently breaking his back to extract.

He only knows the conversion rate: One sack of stones equals one bowl of cassava. Two sacks equal safety for another day.

This disconnection creates a unique psychological state known as **Alienated Labor**, but in a war zone, it is far more toxic. Michel is not just a worker; he is a tool. He has been objectified.

When a human being is treated as a machine for years, the brain begins to accept this definition. This is **Dehumanization** but internalized. Michel does not view his body as "himself." He views his arms as levers and his back as a load-bearing beam. If he feels pain, he ignores it, not out of bravery, but because machines do not feel pain. He has dissociated from his own biology to survive the labor.

III. The Architecture of Moral Injury

The mine is controlled by a militia group. They are men who wear mismatched fatigues and sunglasses, carrying AK-47s that look cleaner than the children.

Six months ago, Michel was in school. He liked history. Then the men came to his village. They burned the school. They took the boys.

This brings us to the core clinical theme of this chapter: **Moral Injury**.

PTSD is based on *fear*—the threat to one's life. Moral Injury is based on *shame*—the violation of one's conscience.
It happens at 2:00 PM. A smaller boy, perhaps eight years old, collapses. He is sliding down the mud wall, the sack of stones

crushing him. He cannot stand up.

The commandant nearest them shouts. He racks the slide of his rifle. He points at Michel.

"You," the commandant barks. "Get him up. Or you take his load too."

Michel freezes. His moral compass, built by his mother and his church, screams: *Help him. Carry his load. Protect the weak.*
But his survival brain screams: *If you take his load, you will collapse. If you collapse, you will die.*
Michel walks over to the boy. He does not help him up. He kicks him.

"Get up!" Michel shouts, mimicking the tone of the guard. "Get up, stupid!"

He kicks the boy again, harder, until the boy cries and scrambles to his feet.

IV. The Fracture of the Soul

In that moment, something inside Michel breaks. It is a fracture more severe than a broken bone.

By kicking the boy, Michel has committed a **Transgression against the Self**. He has violated his own definition of what it means to be a "good person."

This creates **Toxic Shame**. Unlike guilt ("I *did* something bad"), shame says ("I *am* bad").

Clinical studies on child soldiers and forced laborers in the Congo show that this is the hardest wound to treat. A child can recover from being beaten. But how does a child recover from being the beater?

Michel returns to his spot. He slams the rebar into the wall.

Thwack.

He hates the commandant. But he hates himself more. The militia has achieved the ultimate victory: they have installed a copy of themselves inside Michel's head. He is now policing himself. He has become the aggressor to survive the aggressor.

V. The Night and the "Shadow"

Night falls over the camp. The boys are herded into a fenced enclosure. They eat their cassava paste with dirty fingers.

Michel sits apart from the others. He looks at his hands. In the dim light of the cooking fires, they look like claws.

He remembers his mother's voice calling him for dinner. The memory feels like it belongs to a stranger. That "Michel" is dead. The Michel who exists now is a creature of the pit.

This is the psychological concept of the **Shadow Self**, adapted from Jungian psychology. The war forces the child to bury their compassion, their gentleness, and their vulnerability deep into the unconscious, because those traits are liabilities. They cultivate a "War Persona"—hard, cruel, unfeeling.
But the "Good Self" is not gone; it is just haunting him.

Michel closes his eyes. He sees the face of the boy he kicked. The shame washes over him—a hot, prickly sensation in the chest.

To cope, he engages in **Numbing**. He refuses to cry. He shuts down the emotional centers of his brain. If he feels nothing, the shame cannot burn him. He stares at the fire until his eyes dry out. He decides, consciously, to become stone.

VI. The Global Complicity

The tragedy of the Congo is not isolated. It is connected by invisible wires to the rest of the world.

Michel sleeps on the ground. Thousands of miles away, a teenager in New York charges their phone. A businessman in Tokyo checks his email. A mother in London takes a photo.

The electrons flowing through those devices rely on the capacitor made from the stone in Michel's hand.

His trauma is the foundation of our connectivity.

As Michel drifts into a fitful sleep, he does not dream of rescue. He dreams of the mud. He dreams that the mud is rising, filling his mouth, filling his ears, until he is no longer a boy, but just another deposit of mineral waiting to be mined.

He has learned the final lesson of the war: *I am not a person. I am a resource.*

And the resource is running out.

CHAPTER 5: THE ART OF KINTSUGI

Focus: The Science of Repair, Neuroplasticity, and Post-Traumatic Growth

Key Concepts: The Window of Tolerance, Somatic Experiencing, Narrative Exposure Therapy, and the Re-integration of the Self.

I. The Biology of Hope

There is a Japanese art form called *Kintsugi*. When a precious ceramic bowl is broken, the master does not throw the shards away. Nor does he try to glue them back together seamlessly to hide the damage. Instead, he mixes the lacquer with powdered gold. He highlights the cracks. The repaired bowl is considered more beautiful than the original because it has a history. It has survived a fracture.

For decades, psychiatry viewed the traumatized brain as a broken bowl that could never hold water again. We believed that once the neural pathways of fear were paved, they were permanent. We believed that a child like Tariq in Gaza or Michel in the Congo was "ruined."

We were wrong.

The most revolutionary discovery in modern neuroscience is **Neuroplasticity**. The brain is not a static machine; it is a river. It is constantly rewiring itself based on experience. Just as the terror of the siege wired Tariq's brain for hyper-arousal, the experience of safety can wire it for connection. The brain *wants* to heal. It produces a protein called **BDNF (Brain-Derived Neurotrophic Factor)**, which acts like fertilizer for new neurons.

This chapter is not about erasing the war. The war is a fact. This chapter is about moving the war from the "forever present" into the "past." It is about taking the shards of these children's lives and filling the cracks with gold.

To see how this works, we must revisit our children. We must watch them do the impossible work of healing.

II. The Silent Room: Reconnecting

the Speech Center

Subject: Olena (Ukraine)
Intervention: Art Therapy and Narrative Exposure

We return to Olena, the six-year-old in the Kharkiv metro. She has been evacuated to a temporary shelter in Lviv, far from the front lines. The sirens are gone, but she is still silent. She sits in a brightly lit room with a therapist named Dr. Kovalenko.

The problem is neurological. When a child experiences extreme terror, the **Broca's Area** of the brain—the center responsible for speech and language—often shuts down. This is why trauma victims say they are "speechless" or "struck dumb." The horror is trapped in the right hemisphere of the brain (the emotional, visual side) and cannot cross the bridge to the left hemisphere (the logical, linguistic side) to be processed.

Dr. Kovalenko does not ask Olena to talk. Asking a traumatized child to "tell me what happened" is clinically counterproductive; it can re-traumatize them.

Instead, she puts a large sheet of paper on the floor. She places a bucket of paint next to it.

"Draw the fear," Dr. Kovalenko says.

Olena dips her hands in black paint. She smears it violently across the paper. She uses red. She creates a chaotic, swirling mess. She is breathing hard.

This is **Externalization**.

As long as the trauma is inside Olena's head, it is a shapeless, infinite monster. By putting it on the paper, she gives it edges. She gives it a border. She makes it finite.

Dr. Kovalenko points to the black swirl. "What is this?"

"The noise," Olena whispers.

It is one word. But neurologically, it is a triumph. The Broca's Area has flickered back online. She has labeled the affect.

Over the next six weeks, the drawings change. They move from abstract chaos to concrete scenes: the metro, the boots, the rabbit. And finally, she draws herself. In the first drawings, she was tiny, almost invisible. In the final drawing, she is large, standing next to a house with a yellow sun.

She has re-authored her story. She is no longer the victim of the noise; she is the narrator of the picture.

III. The Thaw: Somatic Experiencing

Subject: Tariq (Gaza)

Intervention: Somatic Release and Titration

We find Tariq in a field hospital near the border. He is physically safe, but he is rigid. His shoulders are pulled up to his ears. He walks with a stiff, robotic gait.

Tariq is stuck in the **Freeze Response**.
Dr. Peter Levine, the developer of Somatic Experiencing, observed that in the wild, an impala chased by a cheetah will often "play dead" or freeze. If the impala survives, it will stand up and vigorously shake its body. This "tremoring" discharges the massive amount of energy mobilized for the flight.

Humans have lost this instinct. We rationalize. We hold it in. Tariq has five years of unspent adrenaline trapped in his fascia and muscles. He is a walking pressure cooker.

The therapist, a specialist named Ahmed, does not ask about the drones. He asks Tariq to sit on a yoga ball.

"I want you to push against the wall with your hands," Ahmed says. "Push as hard as you can. Like you are trying to push a truck."

Tariq pushes. His muscles strain. He grunts.

"Harder," Ahmed says. "Feel your arms. Feel your power."

Tariq pushes until his arms begin to shake.

"Good," Ahmed says softy. "Let it shake. Don't stop it."

Tariq's hands tremble. Then his shoulders. Then his torso. He begins to weep, not from sadness, but from release. This is the **Discharge**. The biological energy that was mobilized for the "fight" he never got to fight is finally leaving his body.

Ahmed guides him carefully. If the release is too intense, Tariq might dissociate again. This technique is called **Titration**—releasing the pressure in small, manageable bursts, like opening a soda bottle slowly.

After twenty minutes, Tariq collapses onto a beanbag chair. For the first time in years, his shoulders drop. His breathing deepens. He sleeps for twelve hours straight. He has finally completed the stress cycle.

IV. The Circle: Restoring the Social Engagement System

Subject: Adil (Sudan)
Intervention: Team Sports and Co-Regulation

Adil is in the refugee camp in Chad. The "Void" has left him hollow. He does not trust anyone. He hoards food. He watches the perimeter.

His brain is stuck in a **Sympathetic Dominance** state (fight/flight). To heal, he needs to activate the **Ventral Vagal Complex**—the part of the nervous system that controls social engagement and safety.

The medicine here is not a pill. It is a soccer ball.

A humanitarian group organizes a league. Adil is given a jersey. It is blue. It is too big for him. But when he puts it on, he is no longer "Refugee #4022." He is a "Blue Team Midfielder."

The game requires **Synchrony**. To pass the ball, Adil has to look at another boy's eyes. He has to anticipate his movement. He has to trust that if he passes the ball, it will come back.
Play is the opposite of war. War is rigid; play is fluid. War is about domination; play is about cooperation.

During the game, Adil scores. The team rushes him. They hug him.

For a traumatized child, touch is often a trigger. But in the context of the victory, the touch registers as "Safe." His body is flooded with **Oxytocin**, the bonding hormone. Oxytocin is the chemical antidote to cortisol. It lowers his heart rate.
After the game, the coach, a Sudanese elder named Uncle Hani, sits the boys down. They drink water. They breathe together.

"We are here," Hani says. "We are the Blue Team. We look out for each other."

Adil looks at the boys around him. The "Void" is filled, just a little bit, by the presence of others. He is part of a tribe again. The architecture of his ego begins to rebuild itself around this new identity.

V. The Cleansing: Healing Moral Injury

Subject: Michel (Congo)
Intervention: Ritual, Community Reintegration, and Forgiveness

Michel, the boy who was forced to be a "creuseur" and a tormentor in the coltan mines, faces the hardest road. He is now in a rehabilitation center run by a local NGO.

He believes he is a monster. No amount of talk therapy can convince him otherwise. Logic cannot penetrate toxic shame.

To heal Moral Injury, we need **Ritual**. The brain responds powerfully to symbolic acts of cleansing.

The community elders organize a ceremony. It is based on traditional restorative justice principles, similar to the *Mat Oput* ceremonies in Uganda.

Michel stands in the center of the circle. The villagers are there—not to judge him, but to witness him.

He is asked to hold a heavy stone. "This is what you carried," the elder says. "This is the weight of the mine. This is the weight of what you did to survive. Was it your choice?"

"No," Michel whispers.

"Was it your spirit that did it?"

"No. It was the soldier in my head."

"Then give it back."

Michel walks to a pit dug in the center of the circle. He throws the stone in. The thud echoes.

The elder takes a bowl of water mixed with herbs. He washes Michel's hands—the hands that broke the stones, the hands that hit the other boy.

"These hands are new," the elder says. "The past is in the hole. The boy is here."

This is **Performative Absolution**. It signals to Michel's unconscious mind that he has been re-accepted into the moral universe of his people.

That night, Michel does not sit alone. He eats from the communal bowl. He is not fully healed—the memories will always be there—but the "Shadow" has receded. He understands that he is not what he did. He is who he is becoming.

VI. The Window of Tolerance

The unifying theory behind all these stories is the **Window of Tolerance**.

Imagine a river. When a child is within the banks of the river, they can handle stress. They can learn. They can love. This is the Window.

War pushes children out of the river.

- **Hyper-arousal (Up):** Panic, rage, vigilance (Adil, Tariq).
- **Hypo-arousal (Down):** Numbing, silence, depression (Olena, Michel).

The goal of all these interventions—the art, the shaking, the soccer, the ritual—is to widen the riverbanks. To help the child stay in the flow.

VII. The Myth of Resilience

We often praise children for being "resilient." We say, "Look how strong they are; they bounced back."

This is a dangerous myth. Children do not "bounce back" like rubber balls. They are more like young trees. If you bend a sapling to the ground and hold it there for years, when you let go, it does not snap back to vertical. It grows crooked.

The work described in this chapter is the work of staking the tree. It is the slow, gentle, daily process of supporting the trunk so that it can find the sun again.

It takes years. It requires funding, expertise, and patience. But the science is clear: **Repair is possible.** The mirror is shattered, yes. But if we pick up the pieces with care, we can build a mosaic that reflects a light more complex and brilliant than the original glass ever could.

THE ARCHITECTS OF TOMORROW

I. The Aggregate Memory

We have traveled a great distance in these pages. We have moved from the claustrophobia of the Gaza skyline to the subterranean chill of the Kharkiv metro. We have walked the red dust road to Chad and stood knee-deep in the mud of the Congo.

If you close your eyes now, you can likely see them.

You see Tariq, freezing at the sound of a drone, his body a map of unspent adrenaline.

You see Olena, coloring the sun black because her world has lost its illumination.

You see Adil, staring into the void of the refugee camp, trying to remember the face of a father who has become a ghost.

You see Michel, looking at his calloused hands, struggling to believe they can ever hold anything other than a weapon or a stone.

These are not four separate stories. They are a single story. They are the **Global Cohort of the Besieged**.

In a polarized world, we are often told to choose sides. We are told that the suffering of one group justifies the suffering of another. But the neurobiology of a child does not have a nationality. A cortisol spike in Ukraine looks identical under a microscope to a cortisol spike in Palestine. The pruning of the prefrontal cortex in Sudan follows the exact same biological script as it does in the Congo.

Pain is the universal language. And right now, it is the loudest language being spoken on Earth.

II. The Epigenetic Clock

The most terrifying aspect of this journey is not what is happening *now*, but what will happen *next*.

We have discussed the concept of **Epigenetics**—the study of how environment alters the expression of our genes. We know that severe trauma can leave a chemical "mark" on the DNA, a mark that can be passed down to the next generation.
If we do not intervene, Tariq's trauma will not end with Tariq. It may live in the anxiety of his daughter. It may live in the autoimmune disorders of his grandson. The war echoes through the bloodline.

We are currently manufacturing a future where millions of adults will be walking around with "survival brains" in a "peacetime world."

- They will be leaders who perceive negotiation as a threat.
- They will be parents who cannot soothe their own children because they were never soothed themselves.
- They will be neighbors who interpret a difference of opinion as a declaration of war.

If we want to know why history repeats itself, this is the answer. It repeats because we sign peace treaties on paper, but we leave the war burning in the neurons of the survivors.

III. The Cost of Looking Away

It is easy to close this book and say, "It is too much. The problem is too big."

That is a defense mechanism. It is your own brain trying to protect you from the pain of empathy. But we do not have the luxury of looking away.

The cost of ignoring these children is not just humanitarian; it is geopolitical. A child who is left in the "Void"—stripped of identity, community, and hope—is the perfect recruit for extremism. When a child feels like *nothing*, they will join any group that promises to make them into *something*.

If we abandon Michel in the mine, we are handing him a rifle. If we leave Adil in the camp for ten years, we are creating a radical.

The most pragmatic investment in global security is not a missile defense system. It is a **Psychosocial Support Program**. It is a school. It is a soccer ball. It is a therapist who sits in the mud and says, "You are still human. You are still good."

IV. The Re-Assembly

So, what is the path forward?

It lies in the title of this book: *The Shattered Mirror*.

When a mirror is shattered, you cannot simply glue it back together and pretend it is new. The reflection will always be fragmented. But you can build a mosaic.

We must build a world that is capable of holding these children. This requires a new kind of architecture—not of buildings, but of systems.

1. **Safety First:** We cannot treat trauma while the bombs are still falling. The cessation of violence is the prerequisite for mental health.
2. **The Witness:** We must stop demanding that children "be resilient" and start demanding that adults be protective.
3. **The Long Haul:** Healing is not a six-week program. It is a twenty-year commitment. It is the work of a generation.

We need "Trauma-Informed" societies. Schools that understand why a refugee child can't sit still. Police forces that understand why a war-torn teenager runs when he sees a uniform. Doctors who ask, "What happened to you?" instead of "What is wrong with you?"

V. A Final Portrait

Imagine a field. It is neutral ground. The soil is rich.

In this field, the drone does not fly. The siren does not wail.

Tariq is there. He is sleeping under a tree, and his sleep is deep and dreamless.

Olena is there. She is painting, and she is using the color yellow.

Adil is there. He is shouting, not in anger, but to call for a pass in a game of football.

Michel is there. He is holding a book, not a stone. His hands are clean.

This place does not exist yet. It is a blueprint. It is a fragile, impossible dream. But it is the only dream worth having.

These children have done the hardest work already. They have survived. They have carried the weight of the sky, the depth of the earth, the heat of the desert, and the darkness of the mine. They are still standing.

They are the architects of the twenty-first century. But they cannot build the house alone. They are waiting for us to pass them the bricks.

They are waiting for us to look into the shattered mirror and see, not a monster, and not a victim, but the reflection of our own shared, fragile, and tenacious humanity.

The war is the injury.

The child is the survivor.

The repair is up to us.

PART II: THE EROSION
"It is not the shock that kills the spirit; it is the duration."

CHAPTER 6: THE CLASSROOM OF DUST

Location: Khan Younis, Gaza Strip

Timeline: Six months into the siege

Subject: Tariq, now Age 10

Clinical Focus: Cognitive Decline, Malnutrition, and the Loss of "Future Orientation"

I. The Hunger of the Mind

Time in the siege does not move in a line; it moves in a circle.

Six months have passed since we first met Tariq. He is ten years old now, technically. But if you were to look at a chart of his developmental milestones, the line would not be going up. It would be flatlining.

Tariq sits on a plastic crate in what used to be a UNRWA school courtyard. The school itself—the concrete structure with the blue logo—is a shell. The west wall is gone, exposing the classrooms like a dollhouse sliced open.

There are no books. There are no desks. There is only the dust.

Tariq is thinner. The frantic energy he had in Chapter 1—the aggression, the shoving at the water truck—has vanished. It has been replaced by a terrifying stillness. He sits for hours, staring at a patch of ground, tracing patterns in the dirt with his toe.

This is the clinical manifestation of **Conservation Withdrawal**.

When an organism realizes that no amount of energy expenditure will change the outcome (he cannot fight the drone; he cannot find more food), the brain initiates a metabolic shutdown. It is a biological hibernation. Tariq is conserving his glucose for the vital organs: heart, lungs, brainstem. The "luxury" functions—curiosity, play, learning, laughter—have been switched off to save power.

II. The Physiology of Starvation

We must address the biology of his silence. Tariq is eating, on average, 600 calories a day. A growing ten-year-old boy requires

1,800.

He is not just hungry; he is suffering from **Micronutrient Deficiency**. Specifically, he is lacking Iron and Zinc.

- **Iron:** Essential for carrying oxygen to the brain. Without it, Tariq is in a constant state of "brain fog." He feels dizzy when he stands up. His thoughts are sluggish, like wading through syrup.
- **Zinc:** Essential for mood regulation and memory.

Inside his hippocampus (the memory center), the neurons are literally shrinking. The dendrites—the little branches that reach out to connect with other neurons to form new ideas—are retracting. Tariq is not just "missing school"; his biological capacity to learn is being dismantled. If you tried to teach him multiplication right now, his brain would struggle to encode it. The hardware is compromised.

III. The Phantom School

Despite the ruins, the adults try to maintain the fiction of normalcy. A volunteer teacher, Mr. Walid, stands before a group of thirty boys sitting on the rubble.

Mr. Walid is gaunt. His suit jacket is covered in gray dust. He holds a piece of chalkboard that was salvaged from the wreckage.

"Today," Mr. Walid says, his voice raspy, "we will talk about the history of trade routes in the Mediterranean."

Tariq watches Mr. Walid's mouth move. He tries to listen. He knows he should care about trade routes. He used to be the top student in geography.

But the words do not stick. They slide off his mind.

Instead, Tariq is focusing on Mr. Walid's pocket. There is a bulge there. *Is it a date? Is it a piece of bread?*

Tariq's entire cognitive horizon has shrunk to the immediate biological imperative. This is the **Loss of Future Orientation**.

To learn history is to believe in a continuum of time. To learn math is to believe you will one day build something. But Tariq no longer believes in "next year." He does not even believe in "tonight." The concept of the future has been amputated by the trauma. Why memorize trade routes if the roof might collapse in an hour?

Mr. Walid asks a question. "Who can tell me what the Phoenicians were famous for?"

Silence. The thirty boys stare blankly. It is not defiance. It is exhaustion. The collective IQ of the group has been temporarily depressed by the trauma load.

Mr. Walid lowers the chalk. He looks at the boys. He sees the glazed eyes. He sees the "thousand-yard stare" on ten-year-old faces.

He drops the chalk. It breaks on the concrete. He sits down on the rubble and puts his head in his hands. The lesson is over.

IV. The Economy of Survival

Tariq leaves the "school." He walks back to his family's tent.

The streets have changed. Six months ago, there was panic. Now, there is a grim, silent economy.

He passes a group of men trading. Money has become useless; the currency is now items of survival. A pack of diapers trades for a bag of flour. A fully charged power bank is worth more than gold.

Tariq has a job. His job is to find combustible material. The gas ran out months ago. To boil water, they need fire.

He enters the shell of a bombed-out apartment building. He

knows this is dangerous—there could be unexploded ordnance (UXO)—but his fear response has been blunted by the routine.

He finds a wooden chair leg sticking out of a pile of masonry. He pulls at it. It is stuck.

He pulls harder. He grunts. The dust makes him cough—a dry, hacking cough that rattles his small chest. The air in Gaza is filled with **particulate matter** from pulverized concrete, asbestos, and heavy metals from munitions. Tariq is breathing in a toxic cocktail that is scarring his lung tissue.

Finally, the wood comes loose. He holds it like a trophy.

Then, he sees it.

Under the rubble where the chair leg was, there is a shoe. A child's sneaker. Blue, with a white stripe.

Tariq knows that shoe. It belonged to his cousin, Bassem. Bassem's building was hit three weeks ago. They never found him.

Tariq stands there, holding the piece of wood. A normal reaction would be to scream, to run, to cry.

Tariq does none of these things. He stares at the shoe. He feels a strange detachment, a numbness spreading from his chest to his fingertips.

"Hello, Bassem," he whispers.

He does not try to dig. He knows he cannot move the slab. He places the piece of wood in his bag. He turns around and walks away.

This is **Emotional Anesthesia**. To survive the intolerable, Tariq has severed his emotional nerve endings. He cannot afford to grieve Bassem right now. If he starts crying, he might not stop, and he needs to get the wood home to boil the water. The pragmatism of survival has cannibalized his humanity.

V. The Night of the Generators

He returns to the tent. His mother, Amira, is there. She looks twenty years older than she did in Chapter 1. Her hair is graying.

She takes the wood. She does not ask where he got it. She does not hug him. She is too tired.

This is the **Erosion of Maternal Attunement**. In the beginning, mothers held their children constantly. Now, the mothers are hollowed out. They are functioning on autopilot. The emotional bond—the "mirror"—is clouding over.

Night falls. The drone hums—the ever-present Zanana.

Tariq lies on the thin mattress. His stomach cramps. It is a sharp, twisting pain. Hunger pangs.

He closes his eyes, but he does not sleep. He enters a state of **Hyper-vigilant Dozing**.

He thinks about the shoe. The image of the blue sneaker loops in his mind. *Blue shoe. Dust. Blue shoe. Dust.*

This is an **Intrusive Thought Loop**. It is a hallmark of complex trauma. The brain gets stuck on a horrifying image like a scratched record.

To stop the image, Tariq does something new. He starts to count.

"One, two, three, four..."

He counts the seconds between the hum of the drone. He counts the beats of his own heart.

He discovers that if he counts, the shoe goes away.

"Four hundred and one... four hundred and two..."

He is developing **Obsessive-Compulsive tendencies** (OCD) as a coping mechanism.

In a world of total chaos, counting is the only thing he can control. It is a desperate attempt to impose order on a disordered universe.

He counts until the numbers blur. He counts until the sun rises, gray and choked with smoke, over the broken city. He has survived another night, but a little less of Tariq is left in the morning.

CHAPTER 7: THE COLD CONCRETE (UKRAINE)

Location: Lviv, Western Ukraine (Displaced)

Timeline: Eight months post-invasion

Subject: Olena, now Age 7

Clinical Focus: Survivor's Guilt, Integration Trauma, and the "Double Life"

Transitioning from the static hunger of Gaza to the confusing safety of displacement in Ukraine.

I. The Safety That Feels Like Danger

Olena is no longer in the metro. She and her mother, Iryna, have been evacuated to Lviv, a city in the west that is relatively safe.

They live in a gymnasium that has been converted into a shelter. It is warm. There are hot meals. There are volunteers who give her candy.

By all logical metrics, Olena should be better. But she is worse.

In the metro, everyone was afraid. The fear was shared. Here, in Lviv, people are walking to cafes. Trams are running. Teenagers are laughing.

This normalcy is terrifying to Olena.

She walks down the street with her mother. A tram rumbles past. Olena throws herself onto the pavement, covering her head.

Passersby stop and stare. A woman looks at her with pity.

Olena stands up, brushing the dirt off her knees. She sees the pity in the woman's eyes, and she feels a surge of hot, white rage.

"Don't look at me!" she screams.

Iryna grabs her hand. "Olena, shh."

"They don't know!" Olena yells, pointing at the people in the cafe. "Why are they drinking coffee? The rockets are coming!"

This is the **Disconnect of the Survivor**. Olena cannot bridge the gap between her internal reality (war) and the external reality (peace). She feels isolated by her trauma. She feels that the "safe" people are naive, or worse, that they are lying.

II. Survivor's Guilt in a Seven-Year-Old

That night, on her cot in the gymnasium, Olena whispers to her mother.

"Mama?"

"Yes, baby."

"Is Grandma still in Kharkiv?"

"Yes. She is too old to travel."

Olena is quiet for a long time. "Is she cold?"

"Maybe a little."

"I have a blanket," Olena says. "I have two blankets."

"That is good."

"It's not good!" Olena starts to cry. "Why do I have two? I should be there. I should be cold too."

This is **Survivor's Guilt**. It is rare to see it so clearly in a child this young, but war accelerates emotional development. Olena feels that her safety is a betrayal. By being warm, she is abandoning her grandmother.

She kicks off her blankets. She lies in the cold air.

"Olena, put your covers on," her mother chides.

"No," Olena says stubbornly. "I want to be cold."

This is **Self-Punishment**. Olena is engaging in a penance ritual. If she suffers physically, she feels less guilty psychologically. She is trying to align her body with the suffering of those she left behind.

III. The Two Olenas

To cope with this dissonance, Olena splits in two.

There is **Day Olena**. She goes to the temporary school. She is quiet. She follows the rules. She says "thank you" to the volunteers. She is the "Good Refugee."

Then there is **Night Olena**. In her dreams, she is back in the metro. But in the dreams, she is not a child. She is a soldier. She is fighting the monsters. She wakes up sweating, thrashing, sometimes screaming profanities that a seven-year-old should not know.

Dr. Kovalenko, the therapist we met briefly in the previous outline, observes this. She notes in her file: *"Subject exhibits marked dissociation between social presentation and internal emotional landscape. The 'False Self' is performing normalcy to avoid burdening the mother."*

Olena is protecting her mother. She sees how fragile Iryna is. So, Olena pretends to be okay. She becomes a **Parentified Child**. She suppresses her own terror to stabilize the family unit.
She draws a picture for her mother. It is a picture of flowers.

"Look, Mama," she says, forcing a smile. "Spring."

She does not draw the roots of the flowers, which in her mind, are growing out of the bones of the dead. She keeps that part to herself. She is seven years old, and she has learned the hardest lesson of the adult world: how to hide the truth to protect the ones you love.

CHAPTER 8: THE WOLF OF THE CAMP

Location: Adré Refugee Camp, Chad Border

Timeline: Eleven months post-displacement

Subject: Adil, Age 12

Clinical Focus: Instrumental Aggression, Conduct Disorder as Survival Strategy, and the Hyper-Arousal of Resource Guarding

I. The City of White Plastic

To understand who Adil has become, you must first understand the city he inhabits.

Adré is no longer a temporary stopover. It has metastasized into a sprawling, chaotic metropolis of white tarpaulin and red dust. It is a city without plumbing, without electricity, and without police. It is a city where the sun is an enemy that rises at 6:00 AM to bake the earth to a cracking point, and where the wind is a weapon that sandblasts the skin.

Adil is twelve now. In the timeline of his body, he has grown two inches. In the timeline of his mind, he has aged a decade.

He walks through Sector D with a gait that is not his own. In Khartoum, he walked with the bouncy, distracted energy of a student. Now, he walks with his center of gravity low, his shoulders hunched forward, his eyes scanning the periphery. It is the walk of a predator in territory that does not belong to him.

He is wearing a t-shirt that says "Paris Saint-Germain," but the logo is peeling, and the fabric is stiff with sweat and grime. He does not care about the shirt. He cares about what is tucked into the waistband of his shorts: a sharpened piece of flattened metal, salvaged from a corned beef tin.

He does not intend to use it. But he knows that *having* it changes the way he stands. It changes the way others look at him. In the camp, the perception of lethality is the only currency that matters.

II. The Politics of the Pump

It is 10:00 AM. The heat is already shimmering off the ground in waves. Adil heads to the water distribution point.

THE SHATTERED MIRROR

This is the town square of the camp. It is also the coliseum.

There are four taps for six thousand people. The line stretches for half a mile. But there is a second line—a shorter, darker line near the front. This is for the "Shabab"—the youth gangs who have enforced a tax on the water.

Adil does not join the back of the line. He walks to the front.

A year ago, Adil would have waited. He would have held his mother's hand. He would have been polite. But the boy who was polite died of thirst three months ago.

He approaches a woman near the front. She is old, her face a roadmap of wrinkles. She is holding two yellow jerrycans.

"Move," Adil says. His voice is flat. It is not a shout; it is a statement of fact.

"have been here since dawn," the woman says, clutching her cans. "Please, son."

"Move back," Adil repeats. He steps closer. He does not threaten her. He simply invades her personal space, projecting a kinetic potential for violence. He taps the metal in his waistband—a subtle, almost invisible gesture.

The woman looks at his eyes. She sees the flatness there. She sees that he has turned off his empathy switch.

She steps back.

Adil places his can under the tap. He fills it. He drinks deep, gulping mouthfuls of the tepid, chlorinated water. He wipes his mouth. He does not look at the woman.

Clinical Insight: Instrumental Aggression

To the outside observer, Adil is a bully. A psychiatrist from the West might diagnose him with Conduct Disorder (CD), characterized by a lack of empathy and violation of social norms.

But this diagnosis fails to account for context. In a war zone, empathy is a caloric expense that the brain cannot afford. Adil's aggression is not "maladaptive"; it is **Instrumental Aggression**. It is a tool used to achieve a specific goal (water).

His brain has learned a new reward loop:
- **Stimulus:** Thirst/Hunger.
- **Action:** Aggression/Dominance.
- **Reward:** Survival.
- **Reinforcement:** The Dopamine hit of success.

Adil is not "bad." He is an efficient biological machine operating in an environment where "goodness" results in death.

III. The Pack

Adil leaves the pump and heads to the edge of the camp, where the tents give way to open scrubland. This is the territory of "The Wolves."

They are a group of six boys, aged ten to fourteen. They are not friends in the way children in peace are friends. They do not share secrets or dreams. They share intelligence.
- *Where is the new aid truck coming from?*
- *Which NGO is handing out high-energy biscuits?*
- *Which sector has the lax security tonight?*

The leader is Musa, a fourteen-year-old with a scar running through his left eyebrow. Musa was a child soldier in Darfur before he fled. He knows how to strip an AK-47, though he doesn't have one here.

"Adil," Musa nods.

"Musa."

They sit in the shade of a thorn bush. They do not play. They plan.

"The MSF truck is coming at 2:00," Musa says. "They have Plumpy'Nut (a peanut-based paste for malnutrition). But they are watching the lines."

"We create a diversion," Adil says. It is the first time he has spoken in an hour.

The plan is simple. Two of the smaller boys will start a fight near the entrance. While the guards are distracted breaking it up, Adil and Musa will slip under the back canvas of the truck.

Clinical Insight: The Gang as a Surrogate Family

Adil's father is missing. His mother is in the tent, incapacitated by depression and heatstroke. He has lost his "Vertical Attachment" (parent-child). So, he replaces it with a "Horizontal Attachment" (peer-to-peer).

The gang provides **Safety in Numbers**. But it demands a price: **Groupthink**. To belong to the pack, Adil must suppress his individual conscience. He cannot be the "son of a pharmacist" anymore. He must be a Wolf. If he shows weakness, the pack will turn on him. This constant performance of toughness creates a thick armor around his ego, making it nearly impossible for him to be vulnerable, even with his own mother.

IV. The Heist

At 2:00 PM, the white Land Cruiser arrives. Dust billows. The crowd surges forward. Desperation has a smell—it smells of sour sweat and old clothes.

Adil watches. His heart rate drops. This is paradoxical. Most people's hearts race before a crime. But Adil is experiencing **The**

Calm of the Hunt. His focus narrows.

"Now," Musa signals.

The two small boys, Ali and Samer, start shoving each other near the bumper. "Thief! He took my card!" Ali screams.

The MSF guards, well-meaning volunteers in vests, rush to separate them. "Hey! Stop! No fighting!"

In that split second of chaos, Adil moves. He is fast. He is liquid. He drops to his belly and slithers under the chassis of the truck. The heat from the exhaust pipe burns his cheek, but he doesn't flinch.

He reaches up, slashing the canvas with his metal shard. A box falls out.

He grabs it. It is heavy.

"Go!" Musa hisses from the other side.

Adil scrambles out, clutching the box to his chest. He sprints. He does not look back. He hears a shout behind him—"Hey! You!"—but it is just noise.

He runs until his lungs burn. He runs until the tents blur into a white tunnel. He reaches the gully, their meeting point.

He drops the box. He rips it open.

It is not Plumpy'Nut. It is medical supplies. Bandages. Iodine. Gauze.

Musa kicks the dust. "Useless."

Adil stares at the bandages. A memory flashes in his mind—his father, the pharmacist, wrapping a cut on Adil's knee. *"Clean it first, Adil. Always clean it."*

For a second, the armor cracks. He feels a wave of nausea. He has stolen medicine meant for the sick. He has stolen from people trying to help him.

"We can sell it," Adil says quickly, covering the crack. "The men in

Sector A will buy the iodine."

"Good," Musa says. He claps Adil on the shoulder. "You are thinking like a man."

Adil smiles. But the smile does not reach his eyes. He feels the dopamine rush of the approval, but underneath it, he feels a cold, hollow ache. He is selling his father's trade. He is selling the very thing his father stood for.

V. The Extinction of the Soft Self

That night, Adil returns to his mother's tent. He has traded the iodine for a small bag of sorghum and a bottle of cooking oil.

His mother, Fatima, is lying on the mat. She looks at the food.

"Where did you get this, Adil?" she asks weakly.

"I found it," Adil lies.

"Adil... did you steal?"

"No," he says. His voice is hard. "I did business."

"Adil, look at me."

He looks at her.

"You are changing," she whispers. "Your eyes... they are hard."

"The world is hard, Mama," he says. He starts to make a fire. "Eat. If you don't eat, you die. I won't let you die."

He is engaging in **Parentification**. He has become the provider. He views his mother's morality as a weakness, a luxury from a time when they had walls and a refrigerator. He feels contempt for her softness, even as he loves her.

Later, while his mother sleeps, Adil sits by the dying embers of the fire.

He pulls out the flattened metal shiv. He sharpens it against a rock. *Scrape. Scrape. Scrape.*

He tries to remember his math tables. Seven times seven is forty-nine.

He tries to remember the capital of France. Paris.

He tries to remember the feeling of his bed in Khartoum.

But the memories are fading. They feel like a movie he watched a long time ago. The only reality is the hunger in his belly, the metal in his hand, and the knowledge that tomorrow, he will have to fight for water again.

He lies down. He does not curl up like a child anymore. He sleeps on his back, one hand on the metal, ready to spring.

The boy who loved math is gone. The Wolf has taken his place.

And the terrifying truth is this: The Wolf is better at surviving.

CHAPTER 9: THE ALGORITHM OF FEAR (GAZA)

Location: Rafah, Southern Gaza

Timeline: Nine months into the siege

Subject: Tariq, Age 10

Clinical Focus: Pattern Recognition, Superstition, and the Dopamine-Cortisol Loop

We return to Tariq to witness how the "Erosion" has affected his cognitive processing.

I. The Mathematician of Death

If Adil has become a Wolf, Tariq has become a Calculator.

Survival in Gaza is not about strength; it is about probability. It is about understanding the algorithm of the airstrikes.

Tariq sits on the roof of a half-collapsed building. He has a notebook. It is filled with data points.
- *Strike at 14:00 (F-16).*
- *Strike at 16:30 (Drone missile).*
- *Strike at 02:00 (Naval artillery).*

He is trying to find the pattern. He believes that if he can crack the code, he can save his family.

This is **Magical Thinking**. It is a common psychological defense in helpless situations. The human brain cannot accept randomness. It cannot accept that death is a roll of the dice. So, it invents patterns.

"If I step on the cracks in the pavement, the bomb will fall," Tariq thinks. So he walks on his tiptoes.

"If I hold my breath for fifty seconds, the drone will turn away." So he holds his breath until he passes out.

He is building a cage of superstitions to hold back the chaos.

II. The Screen Addiction

Tariq is not just watching the sky; he is watching a screen. He has inherited his older brother's phone. He spends every waking hour scrolling through Telegram channels that track the strikes.

"Red Alert: Activity over Khan Younis."

"Photo: Smoke rising near the hospital."

He scrolls. He refreshes. He scrolls.

This is **Doomscrolling**, but on a pathological level.
Every time he sees a notification, his brain gets a hit of **Cortisol** (fear). When he confirms the strike is *not* near him, he gets a hit of **Dopamine** (relief).

This cycle—Terror/Relief, Terror/Relief—is chemically addictive. Tariq is addicted to his own fear. If the phone runs out of battery, he goes into a panic attack. Not because he is in danger, but because he has lost his connection to the "control center."

III. The Dissolution of the Mirror

One afternoon, Tariq is showing his notebook to his uncle.

"Look," Tariq says, pointing to his charts. "They never strike between 3:00 and 3:15. It is the shift change."

His uncle looks at the scribbles. They are nonsense. Just random times and lines.

"Tariq," his uncle says gently. "Put the book away. Go play."

"It's not a game!" Tariq screams. He throws the book. "I am saving us!"

He runs away. He hides in a small concrete pipe.

He catches his reflection in a puddle of sewage water. He looks at his own face.

For a moment, he does not recognize himself. The eyes staring back are too old. The mouth is set in a permanent grimace.

This is **Depersonalization**. He feels like he is a pilot controlling a robot body. The "Tariq" who liked cartoons is floating somewhere above him, watching this dirty, angry boy in the pipe.

He splashes the water, destroying the reflection. He prefers the ripples. He prefers the distortion. Because looking at the truth—that he is a ten-year-old boy who cannot stop an F-16 with a notebook—is too terrifying to endure.

CHAPTER 10: THE IRON PUBERTY

Location: Rubaya, North Kivu, DRC

Timeline: Fourteen months later

Subject: Michel, Age 14

Clinical Focus: Adolescent Brain Development, Testosterone & Aggression, and the "Truncated Future"

I. The Chemical Storm

Michel is fourteen. In a peaceful country, this is the age of the voice crack, the first awkward shave, the rebellion against parents, and the dizzying, terrifying rush of first attraction. It is a time when the brain is pruning itself to prepare for independence.

But Michel is standing waist-deep in a pit of gray slurry, holding a shovel that weighs fifteen pounds.

His body is changing. He has grown three inches in the last year. His shoulders have broadened, the muscles ropy and hard under skin that is permanently stained with mineral dust.

Inside his body, a chemical war is being fought.

The Clash of Hormones

On one front, Testosterone is flooding his system. It is driving the growth of muscle mass and deepening his vocal cords. It is also driving the urge for dominance, status, and risk-taking.

On the other front, Cortisol (stress) is still at flood-stage levels.

In a normal adolescent, the **Limbic System** (emotion/drive) matures faster than the **Prefrontal Cortex** (impulse control). This is why teenagers are moody and reckless. But in Michel, the gap is catastrophic. His "gas pedal" (testosterone/limbic) is floored, but he has no "brakes" (prefrontal cortex/safety). The trauma has arrested the development of his regulatory systems.

He feels a constant, simmering rage. It is not the helpless fear of the child he was a year ago. It is a hot, pressurized desire to break something. To hit back. To assert that he exists.

II. The Economy of the Body

The *commandant*, a man named Silas, notices the change.

A year ago, Michel was a "rat"—small enough to crawl into the narrowest tunnels. Now, Silas looks at Michel's arms. He sees leverage. He sees torque.

"You," Silas says, pointing with his cigarette. "No more tunnels. You carry the sacks."

This is a promotion. The "carriers" are the mules of the mine. They haul fifty-kilogram sacks of ore up the slippery mud banks to the washing stations.

Michel hoists the sack. His knees buckle, then lock. He grunts. He forces his legs to move.

Clinical Insight: The Body as Capital

Michel realizes something profound and terrible: My value has increased.

In the logic of the mine, his body is a machine. A bigger engine means more output. He feels a perverse pride in this. When he reaches the top of the hill, sweating and panting, he looks down at the younger boys—the "rats"—with a sneer.

He is identifying with his own exploitation. He is becoming proud of his ability to suffer. This is a psychological defense called **Overcompensation**. If he can be the strongest mule, the hardest worker, then maybe he is not a victim. Maybe he is a king.

III. The Risk Calculus

Adolescence is the golden age of risk-taking. Nature designed it this way so that young men would leave the safety of the tribe to hunt and find mates.

In the mine, this instinct is weaponized.

It is raining hard. The pit walls are unstable. A rational adult would stop digging. A fearful child would hide.

But Michel is fourteen. He is high on adrenaline and the toxic masculinity of the militia camp.

"I bet I can get a full sack from the lower vein before the wall slips," he boasts to a friend, Jean.

"You're crazy," Jean says. "It's sliding."

"Watch me."

Michel jumps into the pit. The mud sucks at his boots. He digs frantically. The wall above him groans—the sound of earth detaching from earth.

He doesn't feel fear. He feels a thrill. This is the **Dopamine-driven Reward System** of the adolescent brain hijacking his survival instinct. He is gambling his life for a moment of status.

He fills the sack. He scrambles out just as a ton of wet clay sloughs off the wall, burying the spot where he stood seconds ago.

He stands on the bank, chest heaving, laughing. It is a manic, jagged sound.

"I am a ghost!" he shouts. " The mud cannot catch me!"

The other boys look at him with awe. In that moment, Michel feels immortal. He has not just survived the death of his childhood; he is courting death like a lover. He is developing an **Addiction to Crisis**. Without the rush of near-death, he feels empty. Peace, if it ever came, would bore him.

IV. The Phantom Woman

That night, in the barracks, the talk turns to girls.

Most of the boys have been in the mines since they were ten. Their understanding of women is fractured. They remember their mothers (a source of grief). And they see the women in the nearby village (a source of shame and longing).

Michel lies on his mat. He tries to conjure an image of a girl. He imagines holding a hand. He imagines a softness.

But the image corrupts. It gets mixed up with the violence he sees every day. The militia men talk about women as spoil—things to be taken, used, and discarded.

Michel hates the militia. But he is swimming in their water. He finds himself thinking thoughts that scare him. *If I am strong, I can take what I want.*

He squeezes his eyes shut. He fights the thought. *No. I am not like Silas. I am not like them.*

But the **Moral Injury** is deepening. The longer he stays in a world where power is the only virtue, the harder it becomes to remember the value of tenderness. He is losing the language of intimacy before he has even learned to speak it. He worries that if he ever touched a girl, his hands would be too rough, his heart too hard. He worries that he would break her, just as he breaks the stones.

V. The Foreshortened Future

A visiting aid worker comes to the camp one week later. She is a woman from Kinshasa, dressed in clean clothes. She is doing a survey.

She stops Michel. "Young man," she says. "How old are you?"

"Fourteen."

"Do you go to school?"

Michel laughs. It is a dry, barking sound. "School is for babies."

"What do you want to be when you grow up?" she asks.

Michel stops. The question hangs in the humid air like a foreign object.

When I grow up.

He tries to look forward. He tries to see five years down the road.

He sees mud. He sees sacks. He sees the rifle he hopes to earn. He sees an early grave in a collapsed tunnel.

He sees nothing else.

Clinical Insight: The Foreshortened Future

Dr. Bessel van der Kolk describes this phenomenon accurately. Trauma destroys the imagination. To plan for the future, you need to feel safe in the present. You need to believe that Time is a benevolent resource.

For Michel, time is an enemy. Time means more pain. Why would he want more of it?

"I will be a *Chef de Colline*," Michel says finally. A hill commander. A warlord.

It is the only example of 'success' he has ever seen.

The aid worker looks sad. She writes something on her clipboard. She sees a tragedy. Michel sees a career path.

He walks away, flexing his calloused hands. He does not know that he has just surrendered his dreams. He only knows that he is hungry, and that the sacks are heavy, and that he is strong enough to carry them.

CHAPTER 11: THE GLASS WALL (UKRAINE)

Location: A High School in Berlin, Germany (Refugee Integration Program)

Timeline: Two years post-displacement

Subject: Katya (Olena's sister), Age 15

Clinical Focus: Social Alienation, Identity Diffusion, and the Burden of the "Good Refugee"

We shift the lens to the teenage girl experience, exploring the psychological toll of fleeing to a "perfect" life in Europe.

I. The Performance of Gratitude

Katya is safe. She is more than safe; she is lucky. She attends a gymnasium in Berlin. The hallways are clean. The teachers are kind. She has a laptop.

She hates it.

She stands in the hallway during break. German teenagers surround her. They are talking about a TikTok trend. They are complaining about a math test. They are laughing about a boy who wore the wrong shoes.

Katya stands behind a **Glass Wall**. She can see them, she can hear them, but she cannot touch their reality.
"Katya, did you see the video?" a girl named Lena asks.

"Yes," Katya lies. She smiles. It is a practiced, brittle smile.

She is exhausted by the **Performance of Gratitude**. Everyone tells her she should be happy. *You are in Berlin! You are safe!* So she has to perform happiness. She has to say "Thank you" a hundred times a day.
But inside, she is screaming.

How can you care about shoes?

Don't you know my friends in Kharkiv are melting snow to flush the toilet?

This is **Alienation**. Her trauma has aged her. She feels like a forty-year-old woman trapped in a fifteen-year-old's body. She looks at these German boys with their smooth hands and unlined faces, and she feels no attraction. She feels only a distant, maternal pity. They are children. She is not.

II. Identity Diffusion

Who is Katya?

In Ukraine, she was a pianist. She was funny. She was loud.

In Berlin, she is "The Refugee."

That is her label. It precedes her into every room. Teachers treat her with fragile gloves. *Don't upset the refugee.* Boys treat her as an exotic tragedy. *The sad girl from the war.*
She is beginning to lose herself. She is experiencing **Identity Diffusion**.
She stops playing the piano. Why play? The music belongs to the "Before."

She starts skipping class. She takes the U-Bahn to the edge of the city, to the gray concrete blocks that remind her of home. She sits on a bench and smokes cigarettes she stole.

She is looking for a feeling of reality. The safety of Berlin feels like a dream—a soft, suffocating marshmallows dream. She craves the hard edge of reality.

III. The Digital Umbilical Cord

Her phone buzzes. It is Dima, her boyfriend from back home. He is seventeen now. He has stayed behind.

They video call. Dima is wearing fatigues. He looks tired, dirty, and exhilaratingly alive.

"I miss you," Katya says.

"It's loud here tonight," Dima says, grinning. "Big booms."

Katya feels a twist of jealousy. Yes, jealousy. She is jealous that he is there, in the center of the world, while she is here in the margin.

"I hate it here," she whispers. "It's so... quiet."

"Don't be stupid," Dima snaps. "Stay there. Be safe."

He doesn't understand. He has a purpose. He is defending the motherland. She has no purpose. She is just... waiting.

Clinical Insight: The Crisis of Meaning

Adolescence is the search for meaning. War gives Dima a surplus of meaning (survival, defense). Displacement gives Katya a deficit of meaning. She is drifting. This aimlessness is a breeding ground for depression and self-destructive behavior.

She hangs up. She looks at the clean, orderly German street. She wants to smash a window. She wants to break the glass wall. But she doesn't. She adjusts her backpack, puts on her mask of gratitude, and walks back to the school she hates, to learn a language she doesn't want to speak, for a future she cannot imagine.

CHAPTER 12: THE SHRINKING WORLD

Location: Adré Refugee Camp outskirts, Chad

Timeline: Fifteen months post-displacement

Subject: Nia, Age 13 (Adil's neighbor)

Clinical Focus: Sexual Trauma, "Weathering," and the Strategy of Invisibility

I. The Geography of Fear

For Adil (Chapter 8), the camp is a hunting ground. For thirteen-year-old Nia, the camp is a cage.

In the psychology of displacement, space is gendered. For boys, the trauma often manifests as *expansion*—roaming, aggression, claiming territory. For girls, the trauma manifests as *contraction*.

Nia lives in a world that has shrunk to the size of a plastic tarp.

Inside the tent, she is safe, but she is suffocating. Outside the tent, she is prey.

The most dangerous place on earth for Nia is not the front line of the war; it is the stretch of scrubland three miles outside the camp perimeter. This is where the firewood is.

To cook the sorghum, they need wood. To get wood, someone must leave the safety of the UN patrols. The men will not go; if they leave the camp, they are conscripted or killed by the militia. So, the task falls to the women and girls.

Nia prepares for the journey at 5:00 AM. She does not dress to look pretty. She dresses to disappear. She wraps her *tobe* (scarf) tight around her head. She smears ash on her cheeks to dull the shine of her skin. She tries to make herself look old, ugly, or invisible.

This is **Protective Self-Objectification**. Nia has learned that her body is not her own; it is a territory that others might try to conquer. Therefore, she tries to devalue the territory.

II. The Walk

She walks with a group of ten other girls. They link arms. This is a survival strategy: **The Phalanx**.

THE SHATTERED MIRROR

They do not speak. They listen. They are listening for the sound of engines—the Toyota pickups used by the *Janjaweed* militias.

Every step is a calculation of risk.
- *Step:* Is that dust on the horizon?
- *Step:* Is that a man or a bush?

Clinical Insight: The Allostatic Load of Anticipatory Anxiety

Nia has not yet been attacked. But her body is behaving as if she is currently being attacked.

Her heart rate is 120 beats per minute, sustained for the four-hour walk. Her blood pressure is dangerously high for a child. This state of constant, high-alert anticipation creates a phenomenon known as **Weathering**.

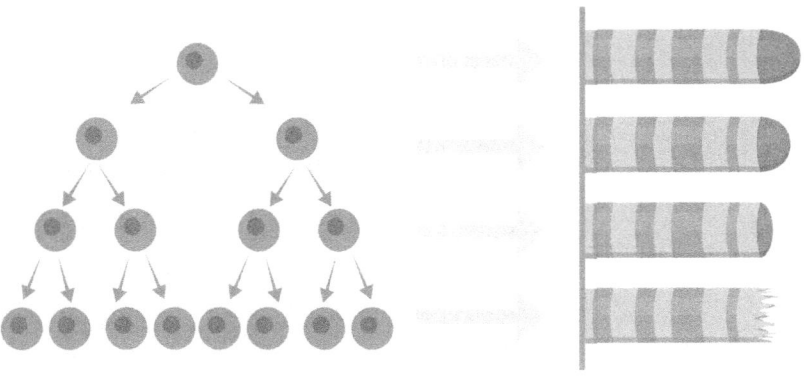

Dr. Arline Geronimus coined this term to describe how chronic social stress causes premature biological aging. Nia's cells are aging faster than a 13-year-old's should. Her telomeres (the protective caps on her DNA) are shortening. If you looked at her

blood markers, she would look like a 40-year-old woman with hypertension. She is being eroded from the inside out, not by what *is* happening, but by what *might* happen.

III. The Transaction

They find the wood. They bundle it quickly, hands shaking.

On the way back, they encounter a checkpoint. It is not the militia this time; it is a local Chadian security post.

The guard is bored. He looks at Nia. He holds his rifle across his chest.

"You can pass," he says, smiling lazily. "But I need a toll."

He does not want money. He touches his crotch.

Nia freezes. The other girls look down.

This is the reality of **Survival Sex** (or Transactional Sex) in conflict zones. It is not prostitution; it is a coercion so systemic it becomes mundane.

Nia has a choice:
1. Refuse, lose the wood, and her family starves (or she is beaten).
2. Pay the "toll."

In this instance, an older woman in the group steps forward. She whispers something to the guard. She hands him a small bag of precious sugar she was hiding. He takes it. He waves them through.

They walk away. Nia feels vomit rising in her throat. She knows that next time, there might not be sugar.

IV. The Bunkerization of the Self

Back in the tent, Nia unloads the wood. Her mother looks at her.

"Did anything happen?"

"No," Nia says.

She lies down in the corner. She pulls her knees to her chest. She covers her head with a blanket.

She is engaging in **Bunkerization**. She is building a wall around her mind. She stops speaking. She stops dreaming. She creates a "Dead Zone" inside herself where she cannot feel fear, but where she also cannot feel love or joy.
Her mother is talking about finding a husband for Nia.

"He is twenty-five," her mother says. "He has a ration card. He can protect you."

In peace, this would be a child marriage, a violation of rights. In war, the logic twists. Marriage is seen as a security strategy. If Nia belongs to one man, perhaps she is safe from the many.

Nia does not argue. She does not care. A husband, a militia, a guard —it is all the same. She has already learned the lesson of the war for women: *You do not exist for yourself.*

CHAPTER 13: THE CHEMISTRY OF THE SOLDIER

Location: Outside Rubaya, DRC
Timeline: Sixteen months later
Subject: Michel, Age 15
Clinical Focus: Desensitization, Substance Abuse, and the Formation of the "Killer Self"

I. The Graduation

We return to Michel. The boy who carried the sacks (Chapter 10) is gone.

He is no longer covered in mud. He is wearing a mismatched uniform: camouflage trousers that are too short, and a black t-shirt. He is holding an AK-47. The wood of the stock is worn smooth.

He has been "promoted" from the mine to the militia.

This transition is not just a change of job; it is a rewiring of the soul. To turn a victim into a killer requires a systematic dismantling of the **Superego** (the conscience).
The militia commanders know this. They do not use logic; they use chemistry and ritual.

II. The Juice and the Powder

Michel's eyes are wide, the pupils dilated to black saucers. He is sweating profusely, though it is a cool night.

He is high.

Before the patrol, the commander gave them "The Juice"—locally brewed alcohol mixed with gunpowder and, sometimes, amphetamines.

Clinical Insight: Pharmacological Disinhibition

The mixture serves a specific neurological purpose.
1. **Alcohol:** Depresses the prefrontal cortex, lowering inhibition and moral judgment.
2. **Amphetamines:** Spike dopamine and adrenaline, creating a sense of invincibility and aggression.
3. **Gunpowder:** Largely placebo but acts as a psychological

totem of magical protection.

Michel feels like a god. The fear that plagued him in the mines is gone, replaced by a buzzing, electric static. He feels a vibration in his teeth. He wants to shoot. Not to kill, necessarily, but just to release the energy trapped in his blood.

III. The Desensitization Sequence

They enter a village. It is suspected of harboring government sympathizers.

The commander points to a hut. "Burn it."

Michel holds the torch. A year ago, the thought of burning a home would have made him sick. Now, he looks at the thatched roof.

He perceives the hut not as a home, but as a target. This is **Reframing**.
He throws the torch. The fire whooshes up.

The dopamine hits him. The fire is beautiful. It is power. For a boy who has felt powerless for two years, the ability to destroy is a seductive drug.

A dog runs out of the burning hut. Another boy, Jean, shoots it. The boys laugh.

Michel laughs too.

This laughter is the sound of **Moral Necrosis**. The tissue of his empathy is dying. He laughs to bond with the group. He laughs to prove he is not weak. He laughs because the drugs tell him it is funny.

IV. The First Kill (The Rupture)

Then, they find a man hiding in the goat pen.

The commander drags him out. He throws him at Michel's feet.

"He is a spy," the commander says. "Finish him."

Michel looks at the man. The man is pleading. He looks like Michel's uncle.

The drugs waver. A crack opens in the armor. Michel's hand shakes. The "Good Boy" inside him wakes up and screams *No*.

"Do it!" the commander roars. He puts a pistol to Michel's head. "Him or you."

This is the **Coercive Rupture**.
Michel pulls the trigger.

The sound is deafening. The recoil hits his shoulder. The man falls.

Michel stands there. His ears are ringing. He waits for the lightning to strike him. He waits for God to stop the world.

But the world continues. The crickets chirp. The fire crackles.

And in that silence, Michel realizes the most terrifying truth of all: *It was easy.*
Physically, pulling a trigger takes less effort than lifting a shovel.

He looks at the gun. It is no longer a heavy weight. It is an extension of his arm.

He has crossed the threshold. He is no longer a civilian. He is a combatant. The **Perpetrator Trauma** has set in. To live with himself, he must now fully embrace the narrative of the militia. He must believe the man was a spy. He must believe the burning was necessary.

He turns to the commander. His face is a mask of stone.

"Where next?" Michel asks.

CHAPTER 14: THE CLASSROOM OF REVENGE

Location: Gaza Strip

Timeline: Two years into the siege

Subject: Tariq, Age 11

Clinical Focus: Radicalization, The "Storehouse of Memory," and Epigenetic Hate

I. The School of Rubble

We return to Gaza. Tariq is eleven. The boy who tried to use math to stop the bombs (Chapter 9) has given up on math.

He has found a new teacher.

He sits in a circle of boys in the ruins of a mosque. The man talking to them is not a schoolteacher like Mr. Walid. He is a younger man, scarred, charismatic. He speaks with a quiet, burning intensity.

"Why do they bomb us?" the man asks.

"Because they hate us," a boy answers.

"No," the man says. "Because they fear us. They know that you are the lions who will take back the land."

Tariq listens. His heart beats faster.

For two years, Tariq has felt like a victim. He has been hungry, scared, and passive. This man is offering him a different story.

He is offering him **Agency**.

Clinical Insight: The Psychology of Radicalization

Radicalization is rarely about religion initially; it is about Dignity.
Tariq feels humiliated. He watches his father beg for flour. He watches his mother cry.
The ideology offers a way to transmute shame into pride. It replaces the painful emotion of "sadness" with the empowering emotion of "rage."

II. The Storehouse of Memory

Tariq goes home. He looks at the wall of their temporary shelter.

On the wall, he has taped pictures. Not of soccer players. Pictures of "martyrs." Men with guns. Men who died fighting.

He looks at the picture of his cousin Bassem (the owner of the blue shoe).

Tariq talks to the picture. "I will not forget you."

This is the **Storehouse of Memory**. In conflict zones, memory becomes a weapon. Forgiveness is seen as a betrayal of the dead. To forget is to kill them a second time.

Tariq is cultivating a **Hostile Attribution Bias**. He interprets every ambiguous event as an act of malice by the enemy.

- The aid truck is late? *They stopped it on purpose.*
- The power is out? *They cut it to punish us.*

This worldview is self-reinforcing. It creates a closed loop where empathy for the "Other" is impossible.

III. The Mirror Neurons Misfire

Tariq watches a video on a phone. It shows a funeral on the "other side"—an Israeli mother crying over her child.

Tariq watches it. He waits to feel sad.

He feels nothing.

"She is acting," he thinks. Or worse: "She deserves it."

This is the failure of the **Mirror Neuron System**. Normally, seeing pain activates the pain centers in our own brain. But Tariq has successfully dehumanized the enemy. His brain categorizes them not as "humans," but as "threats."

He turns off the phone. He picks up a rock. He practices throwing it against a wall.

Thwack.

"One day," he whispers. "Not a rock."

He is not a terrorist. He is an eleven-year-old boy who has been taught that the only way to be a man is to be a avenger. He is the product of a laboratory of suffering that has been running unsupervised for years.

He walks out into the gray light. He looks at the horizon. He does not see a future of peace. He sees a future of fire. And for the first time in two years, he smiles. Because in a future of fire, at least he will be holding the match.

PART III: THE RECLAMATION

"They buried us, but they didn't know we were seeds." — Mexican Proverb

CHAPTER 15: THE UN-DOING

Location: Transit and Orientation Center (CTO), Goma, DRC
Timeline: Three years post-abduction
Subject: Michel, Age 16
Clinical Focus: Chemical Withdrawal, Moral Repair, and the "River of Life" Narrative Therapy

I. The Extraction

Michel does not walk out of the forest; he is carried.

A UN peacekeeping patrol intercepts his militia unit. There is a firefight. Michel, malnourished and high on "The Juice," tries to run, but his body finally revolts. He collapses from malaria and exhaustion.

He wakes up in a white room. It smells of antiseptic—a smell that, to him, is alien and terrifying.

He is in a DDR Center (Disarmament, Demobilization, and Reintegration). He is alive. But he is furious.

He thrashes against the sheets. "Where is my rifle?" he screams. "Give it to me!"

This is not gratitude. This is **Status Withdrawal**. For two years, the rifle was his identity. It was his spine. Without it, he feels naked. He feels like the "rat" in the mine again. He spits at the nurse. He bites the orderly.

He is not a "rescued child" in his own mind. He is a captured soldier.

II. The Chemical Exorcism

The first week is not about psychology; it is about biology. Michel is detoxing.

The mixture of alcohol, gunpowder, and amphetamines has rewired his dopamine receptors. Now that the supply is cut, his brain is crashing.

He sweats through the mattress. He shakes so violently his teeth chatter. He hallucinates. He sees the burning hut. He sees the man he shot standing in the corner of the room, bleeding.

"Go away!" Michel shrieks at the empty corner.

Dr. Kabeya, the center's psychiatrist, watches from the doorway. He knows he cannot talk to Michel yet. The boy's **Prefrontal Cortex** is offline. He is trapped in a **Limbic Storm**.
They treat him with hydration, sedatives, and high-calorie paste. They wait for the chemistry to leave the blood.

III. The Circle of Stone

Three weeks later. Michel is sitting in a circle with twelve other boys. They all look the same: hollow-eyed, jumpy, aggressive.

Dr. Kabeya sits with them. He places a large stone in the center of the room.

"Who is the strongest?" Dr. Kabeya asks.

Michel stands up immediately. "I am."

"Pick up the stone," the doctor says.

Michel picks it up. It is heavy, perhaps twenty kilos.

"Hold it," Dr. Kabeya says. "Do not put it down."

Michel holds it. He smirks. This is a test of strength. He knows how to suffer. He holds it for five minutes. His arms tremble. Ten minutes. His sweat drips onto the floor.

"Put it down," Dr. Kabeya says softly.

Michel drops it. *Thud.*
"How do your arms feel?"

"Light," Michel says.

"This is the anger," Dr. Kabeya says to the group. "It makes you feel strong when you hold it. But it is just a rock. You cannot build a house with it if you are always holding it. You have to put it down to build."

This is **Metaphor Therapy**. These boys have no vocabulary for "trauma" or "PTSD." But they understand weight. They understand burdens.

IV. The River of Life

The core intervention begins a month later. It is called the **River of Life** exercise.

Michel is given a long scroll of paper. He is asked to draw his life as a river.

- **The Source:** His village, his mother, the time before the mine.
- **The Rapids:** The abduction, the mine, the militia.
- **The Ocean:** The future.

Michel draws. He draws the village with green crayons. He draws the mine in black.

But when he gets to the militia part, he stops. He holds the red crayon. He cannot draw the man he shot.

"It is stuck," Michel whispers.

"The river is blocked?" Dr. Kabeya asks.

"Yes. There is a dam. A dead body."

"If the water stops," the doctor says, "it becomes poison. It must flow."

Michel starts to cry. It is not the angry, barking cry of the mine. It is the deep, heaving sob of a child. He draws the red figure. He draws the blood.

"I am bad," Michel says. "I am a devil."

"No," Dr. Kabeya says firmly. "You were a boy in a devil's world. The river flowed through a bad place. But the water is still water."

This is **Externalization of the Problem**. Michel learns to separate his *core self* from the *actions* he was forced to commit. He begins to understand that the "Killer Self" was a costume he wore to survive, not his skin.

V. The First Gentle Touch

The breakthrough happens not in therapy, but in the garden.

Michel is assigned to tend the vegetable patch. He is digging (an action he knows), but this time, he is not digging for coltan. He is planting beans.

He finds a caterpillar on a leaf.

The old Michel—the soldier—would have crushed it. Weakness must be purged.

But Michel stops. He looks at the green, fuzzy creature. He remembers the "River." He remembers that he is "water," not "stone."

He gently moves the caterpillar to another leaf so he doesn't hurt it.

He freezes. He looks at his hands. These are the hands that pulled the trigger. But they just saved a bug.

Clinical Insight: Neuroplasticity in Action

In that moment, a new neural pathway fires.

- **Stimulus:** Vulnerable creature.
- **Old Response:** Kill.
- **New Response:** Protect.

The more he practices this—tending the plants, feeding the center's goat, helping a younger boy tie his shoes—the stronger this pathway becomes. The "Killer Self" is being pruned away, and the "Nurturing Self" is being irrigated.

He is not "cured." The nightmares still come. But he has discovered that his hands can do two things. And for the first time in three years, he chooses the second thing.

CHAPTER 16: THE DEFROSTING

Location: Foster Home, Khartoum, Sudan (Relocated)

Timeline: Two years post-camp

Subject: Adil, Age 14

Clinical Focus: Resource Guarding, Attachment Theory, and the "Safe Surprise"

I. The Hoard

Adil has been lucky. Through a UN reunification program, he was moved out of the camp in Chad and placed with a foster aunt in a stable part of Khartoum (before the new conflict flared).

He lives in a house with walls. There is a refrigerator. There is a tap that produces water whenever you turn it.

But Adil cannot stop being the Wolf.

His aunt, Salma, finds things under his bed.
- Dried crusts of bread.
- Empty water bottles filled with tap water.
- A knife stolen from the kitchen.

Adil is engaging in **Resource Guarding**. His brain does not believe the abundance is real. He expects the famine to return at any second.
He eats too fast. He hunches over his plate, shielding it with his arm. If Salma walks behind him while he eats, he growls—a low, guttural sound in his throat.

II. The War on Safety

Salma is patient. She does not punish him. She understands **Trauma-Informed Care**.
She realizes that "Safety" is a trigger for Adil.
- Chaos feels normal.
- Calm feels suspicious. *When is the blow coming?*

Adil tries to provoke her. He breaks a vase. He yells. He is testing the perimeter. He is asking the silent question: *When will you kick me out? When will you stop loving me?*
He wants her to explode. If she explodes, the world makes sense

again. Violence he understands. Kindness confuses him.

III. The Turning Point: The "Safe Surprise"

One afternoon, Adil is sitting on the floor, guarding his hoard of bread under the bed.

Salma walks in. She holds a tray.

"Adil," she says.

He stiffens. He grips the knife under his pillow.

"I made basbousa," she says. It is a sweet semolina cake.

She puts the tray on the floor. She does not come close. She sits near the door.

"It is too much for me," she says. "Will you help me eat it?"

Adil looks at the cake. It smells like syrup and coconut. It smells like his life before the war.

"Why?" he asks suspiciously.

"Because it is Tuesday," she says. "And because you are here."

She eats a piece. She waits.

Adil crawls out from under the bed. He takes a piece. He eats it.

Then, Salma does something crucial. She pushes the whole tray toward him.

"You can have it all," she says. "And if you finish it, there is more in the kitchen. And more at the store. We will not run out, Adil."

Adil stares at the tray. **Abundance**.

For the first time, his **Amygdala** (threat detector) quiets down, and his **Ventral Vagal System** (social engagement) wakes up.

He does not have to fight for the cake. He does not have to steal it. It is given.

He starts to cry. He cries into the cake.

Salma moves closer. She does not hug him yet—that is too much. She just puts her hand on his ankle. A grounding touch.

"You can sleep, Wolf," she whispers. "The hunt is over."

IV. The Return of Play

Six months later.

Adil is in the courtyard. A neighborhood game of football is starting.

For a year, Adil refused to play. He only watched, calculating threats.

But today, the ball rolls to his feet.

A boy yells, "Pass it!"

The old Adil would have held the ball. Mine.
The Wolf would have popped the ball. Dominance.
The new Adil looks at the ball. He looks at the boy.

He kicks it. A perfect, arcing pass.

He runs. He feels the wind in his hair. He is not running from a militia. He is not running to a food truck. He is running for the sheer, biological joy of motion.

He laughs.

It is a rusty sound, creaky and unsure. But it is there. The **Play Circuit** in his brain, dormant for three years, has flickered back to life.

He is not fully healed. He still checks the locks on the doors three times a night. He still keeps one bottle of water under his bed. But he is no longer a Wolf. He is a boy with a scar, learning how to be a boy again.

CHAPTER 17: THE MOSAIC

Location: A Virtual Classroom (Connecting Ukraine, Gaza, Sudan, Congo)

Timeline: Five years later

Theme: Integration and the "Wounded Healer"

I. The Zoom Call

The world has moved on. The news cameras have left. But the children remain.

We see a screen. It is a video conference for a "Youth Peace Initiative."

- **Top Left:** Michel (19). He is a community organizer in Goma. He helps rehabilitate other child soldiers. He speaks with a quiet authority.
- **Top Right:** Katya (20). She is in university in Berlin, studying International Law. She uses her "Glass Wall" perspective to advocate for refugee rights.
- **Bottom Left:** Adil (19). He is training to be a pharmacist, like his father. He coaches the neighborhood football team.
- **Bottom Right:** Tariq (16).

Tariq is the hardest story. He is still in Gaza. The rebuilding is slow. He is not "cured." He still hates the drones. But he has put down the rock. He is learning coding. He wants to build digital infrastructure that cannot be bombed.

II. Post-Traumatic Growth

They are talking to each other.

"Do you still have the dreams?" Michel asks.

"Sometimes," Katya says. "But I know they are just dreams now."

"I count," Tariq says. "When I get scared, I count."

"I run," Adil says.

They are comparing scars. But they are not competing.

This is the final stage of healing: **Meaning Making**. They have taken the worst things that happened to them and turned them into a source of empathy. They are "Wounded Healers."

They understand something the rest of the world does not. They know the fragility of civilization. And because they know how easily it breaks, they are the most careful builders we have.

III. The Final Image

The book ends not with a period, but with a question mark.

We zoom out from the screen. We see the world. It is still a dangerous place. There are new wars starting today. New children are hearing the siren for the first time.

But we know now that the damage is not the end of the story.

We know that the brain can heal.

We know that the Wolf can become the Boy.

We know that the Stone can become the Water.

The mirror is shattered. The cracks catch the light. It is not perfect. It never will be again. But as the light hits the gold-filled fissures of their lives, it shines with a brilliance that is blinding, defiant, and undeniably, triumphantly human.

The End

SELECTED BIBLIOGRAPHY

I. The Neurobiology of Trauma
(The Body & The Brain)

These texts provide the scientific foundation for the chapters regarding the HPA axis, cortisol spikes, and the physical erosion of the child.

- **Van der Kolk, Bessel.** *The Body Keeps the Score: Brain, Mind, and Body in the Healing of Trauma.* Viking, 2014. (The seminal text on how trauma physically reshapes the brain).
- **Sapolsky, Robert M.** *Why Zebras Don't Get Ulcers.* Henry Holt and Co., 2004. (Essential for understanding the long-term damage of the stress response/cortisol on the immune system).
- **Harris, Nadine Burke.** *The Deepest Well: Healing the Long-Term Effects of Childhood Adversity.* Houghton Mifflin Harcourt, 2018. (Focuses on ACEs—Adverse Childhood Experiences—and physical health outcomes).
- **Levine, Peter A.** *Waking the Tiger: Healing Trauma.* North Atlantic Books, 1997. (The basis for the "Somatic Experiencing" and "Freezing" concepts used in the Gaza/Ukraine chapters).
- **Yehuda, Rachel.** *Epigenetics and the Intergenerational Transmission of Trauma.* World Psychiatry, 2018. (The key research on how trauma marks DNA).

II. Child Development & Attachment
(The Mind of the Child)

These sources support the concepts of the "Good Enough Mother," the "Mirror," and the loss of the future.

- **Perry, Bruce D., and Maia Szalavitz.** *The Boy Who Was Raised as a Dog.* Basic Books, 2006. (Crucial for understanding how trauma affects the developing child's brain and the importance of patterned, repetitive

healing).
- **Winnicott, D.W.** *Playing and Reality.* Routledge, 1971. (Source of the "Holding Environment" and "Transitional Object" concepts used in the Ukraine bunker chapters).
- **Bowlby, John.** *Attachment and Loss (Vol. 1-3).* Basic Books, 1969. (The foundational theory on why separation from the caregiver is the primary trauma).
- **Siegel, Daniel J.** *The Developing Mind: How Relationships and the Brain Interact to Shape Who We Are.* Guilford Press, 2012.

III. The Psychology of War & Political Violence

These texts address the specific contexts of Gaza, Child Soldiers, and Displacement.

- **Jabr, Samah.** *Behind the Frontlines.* Books on Demand, 2018. (Dr. Jabr is a key figure in Palestinian mental health; she argues for the shift from PTSD to "Continuous Traumatic Stress").
- **Boss, Pauline.** *Ambiguous Loss: Learning to Live with Unresolved Grief.* Harvard University Press, 1999. (The core framework for the Sudan chapters—grieving without a body).
- **Honwana, Alcinda.** *Child Soldiers in Africa.* University of Pennsylvania Press, 2006. (Essential reading for the Congo chapters and the concept of "tactical agency").
- **Shay, Jonathan.** *Achilles in Vietnam: Combat Trauma and the Undoing of Character.* Scribner, 1994. (The origin of the term "Moral Injury," applied here to the child combatant).
- **Betancourt, Theresa S., et al.** *Psychosocial adjustment and mental health in former child soldiers in Sierra Leone.* The Lancet, 2010.

IV. The Sociology of Displacement

& Radicalization

Context for the Refugee Camp (Sudan/Chad) and Radicalization (Gaza) chapters.

- **Agamben, Giorgio.** *Homo Sacer: Sovereign Power and Bare Life.* Stanford University Press, 1998. (Philosophical context for the "camp" as a space where rights are suspended).
- **Arendt, Hannah.** *The Origins of Totalitarianism* (specifically the chapter on "The Decline of the Nation-State and the End of the Rights of Man").
- **Geronimus, Arline T.** *Weathering: The Extraordinary Stress of Ordinary Life in an Unjust Society.* Little, Brown Spark, 2023. (Source for the concept of "Weathering" and biological aging in the teenage girl chapter).

V. Recovery & Resilience (The Repair)

Sources for Part III: Healing, Play Therapy, and Narrative Exposure.

- **Frankl, Viktor E.** *Man's Search for Meaning.* Beacon Press, 1946. (The philosophical basis for finding meaning in suffering).
- **Herman, Judith.** *Trauma and Recovery.* Basic Books, 1992. (The three stages of recovery: Safety, Remembrance/Mourning, and Reconnection).
- **Masten, Ann S.** *Ordinary Magic: Resilience in Development.* Guilford Press, 2014. (Debunks the myth that resilience is a superpower; argues it comes from ordinary resources).

Academic Journals Referenced for Data Points:

- *The Lancet Psychiatry* (Global mental health statistics).
- *Journal of Traumatic Stress* (Specific studies on blast waves and acoustic trauma).
- *Social Science & Medicine* (Data on refugee integration).
- *Child Abuse & Neglect* (Data on malnutrition and cognitive decline).

Made in the USA
Coppell, TX
10 January 2026

68833051R00069